The Doctor's Ego

Perennial cause of death and dysfunction in hospitals

Nigel Jack MB ChB FRCA

Foreword - Jörgen Bruhn

I first met Nigel Jack years ago in the day surgery unit of the hospital where he was working. I was impressed how he as an anaesthesiologist not only performed his anaesthesia tasks but also guaranteed a smooth workflow in this busy unit integrating surgeons, nurses and all other health care professionals circling around him. And this all seemingly effortlessly.

At that time I thought it was just due to his outstanding performance in general and regional anaesthesia.

In the next years we both joined the trainer team of the Dutch course for ultrasound-guided regional anaesthesia. Then I realised that it was not about his techniques or his teaching methods. It was about his way of interacting and communicating which made the people flock around him.

When he gave me a first read of one of the first drafts of this book I was blown away.

I was mesmerised by the excellent mixture of deep insight and applied modern communication theory with a charming personal touch by interweaving personal stories and experiences of the author.

Do not underestimate its content and message because of the easy flow of the book. There are more layers than someone might initially think and it points to the secrets of successful communication, interpersonal relationships and meaningful life.

The last chapters are different but not less fascinating: dealing with critical life events, decisions about life and death and its consequences. It is thought provoking, soul shaking and open for controversial opinions.

Read it and use it. After a while re-read it and keep using it.

Then give it to your colleagues, students and residents, and to your friends and family members.

May you and those around you get the maximum benefit out of it.

Jörgen Bruhn, MD PhD

Professor of Anaesthesiology

Nijmegen, 2019

Foreword - Johannes Knape

The Dutch medical training system is internationally highly respected and delivers well qualified doctors for general practice. They are adequately equipped with medical knowledge and techniques. Following the Canmeds principles gives them sufficient training in the areas of co-operation, communication, social skills, education and professional behaviour.

Nonetheless, young specialists (and I speak for my own discipline, anaesthesia, but this certainly also applies to other specialties), particularly at the start of their career, but also later, are confronted with situations in which they are insufficiently prepared or equipped. The change of status from specialist in training to independent medical specialist is different to the daily practice of a collegial group, and more profound than they often anticipate. Also the relationship with specialists in other disciplines demands a different approach. Established power relations and neurotic behaviour by colleagues demand an adequate and proactive answer and attitude from the young medical specialist.

The Doctor's Ego is a book that tackles in particular just these aspects of the work of a medical specialist. This book focuses regularly, and from time to time humorously, on communication from and between specialists and the ways they interact. The effects of large egos, often seen in medical specialists, form an obstruction to good functioning in medical practice. Burnout and work absences are usually not caused by insufficient knowledge or proficiency but by the egos and the friction they cause in communication accompanied by narcissistic, theatrical, neurotic and compulsive behaviour. Even more serious is that these characteristics obstruct the growth of a vital safety culture in healthcare, leading to great damage to quality and patient protection.

The book has been written by a medical specialist with decennia of experience in Dutch practice and with exceptional antennes for human interac-

3

tion and for verbal and non-verbal communication between workers in the health sector.

This book is highly recommended for every starting medical specialist and also for more experienced colleagues as an aid to the fulfilment of a career working in patient healthcare.

Prof. dr. J.T.A. Knape

Emeritus professor of Anaesthesiology University Medical Centre Utrecht
Past-president European Board of Anaesthesiology 2003-2007
Past president European Society of Anaesthesiology 2008-2009.

Preface

This book, written by a medical specialist with more than 40 years experience, was primarily intended to help young doctors avoid many of the pitfalls we encounter daily in our work. It will also be of interest to a wider public, offering real life observations, insights and anecdotes in non-medical language on a wide range of subjects related to medical practice.

Of the many factors determining whether a patient is in good hands, there is probably nothing more influential than the doctor's ego. This book is full of examples to illustrate this and other psychological factors, taken from the author's experience as an anaesthesiologist. Some are light-hearted and some horrifying. The primary focus is on communication and the effects of an oversized ego on patient care. There is a chapter relating the dramatic story of a young woman with chronic pain who was heading inexorably toward death. Another chapter presents the author's arguments for legalising euthanasia, supported by the heart wrenching story of a young woman dying from cancer.

If the subtitle seems melodramatic, just pause to think what the effect is on the survival chances of a patient during a high-risk operation when the surgeon's ego prevents him calling in help from a more experienced colleague. Unlikely? Here's a heading from the Telegraph on 4th August 2018: "Feuding surgeons put patients at risk at heart surgery unit, report finds."

It is the author's hope that junior doctors reading this book will find lessons to help them become more effective and happier professionals. Applying the principals espoused in this book could be life-changing for anyone reading with an open mind.

Introduction

O ver the years I have been fascinated by human interactions, and amazed at how bad some doctors are at communicating. This is to the detriment of their own lives and happiness and the relations with patients and Co-workers, not to mention patient safety.

Because they are near the top of the hierarchy, doctors have a tremendous influence on the atmosphere in a department. For the same reason they are often excluded from accountability, even when they wreck the cohesion of the same department. People in the lower echelons are regularly expected to follow communication courses, whilst the specialists sometimes feel free to show anger, disrespect, and pure rudeness without any correction or consequences. Put simply, doctors get away with behaviour that would lead to the dismissal of a worker without that status, and this behaviour is demonstrated by someone in most hospitals on a daily basis. It's a big problem.

A doctor's career centres around communication; it is their core competence. The lucky ones will have learned healthy and open communication as children. Many are less fortunate; I learned for instance the famous "stiff upper lip" thing. One did not speak of one's feelings. I'm not alone in this, and this is why so many conflicts remain unresolved; people talk at length about the <u>facts</u> of the matter, when the conflict would disappear like snow in many cases if they were to be open about the underlying <u>feelings</u>. "Solve the feelings and you solve the conflict".

As a medical student I learned about the structure of the human inner ear and then did nothing with this knowledge for the next 40 years; if that time had been spent on an aspect of communication, I could have put it to daily use. Neither during my training to be a doctor, nor in my training to become an anaesthesiologist was one single hour spent on communication. Looking back, it seems just as incomprehensible as it then seemed normal. Fortunately times are changing, and more attention is now paid to this aspect. It is in my opinion still not enough.

I do not wish to give the impression that doctors are on average worse communicators than other people; it is just that their profession makes weaknesses in communication glaringly obvious. Although many are empathic and excellent in their patient interactions, it remains a fact that the great majority of complaints against doctors are related to poor communication skills.

I have learned much about communication through the years, and in the recent past I have made a deeper study, including NLP, negotiation theory and Mediation. I have learned how we influence each other, and how unreliable our thought processes and memory can be. I have learned how we tend to over-rate ourselves and how we rationalise the many unkind or silly things we do. One thought pervades: if only I had known this when I was younger! I would then have been a better doctor, a better father and a better husband. I have long hoped that I would have the chance to share some of what I have learned with young colleagues who are at the beginning of their careers. This book is one way to achieve that. It was in large part originally written as a series of letters to someone just starting out on the road to becoming a doctor.

Over the years, I have been as acquisitive of ideas about communication and psychology as any magpie, and in this book I tip my treasure trove onto the table for others to pick and choose. Forgive me for mainly using the "he" form instead of "he or she" for readability. I have to admit that I may be becoming a little old fashioned in a time when the majority of young doctors are women!

Nigel Jack

Anesthesiologist

Heumen, the Netherlands 2019

Anaesthesia is a situation in which the half-asleep watch over the half-awake being half-murdered by the half-witted

Rude Surgeons, Angry patients and

quality

A 2017 study led by Vanderbilt University Medical Centre (VUMC) investigators in collaboration with six other major academic health systems examined data for 32,125 patients from seven academic medical centres, to look at the link between increased patient complaints and risk of medical complications. Put simply, rude surgeons had a 14% higher complication rate than their well behaved peers. The complications included surgical-site infections, pneumonia, kidney conditions, stroke, heart problems, blood clots, sepsis and urinary tract infections. It's perhaps unexpected, but not entirely surprising, and it is certainly worth considering the implications of this finding.

In the study, a man reported getting this response when asking about his wife's upcoming surgery: "Look, your wife will die without this procedure. If you want to ask questions instead of allowing me to do my job, I can just go home and not do it."

One of the major consequences is the estimated cost to health services - 350.000 extra complications per year in the U.S. alone, costing more than three billion dollars. That's a serious amount of money that could be put to better ends than cleaning up behind naughty doctors.

Among the explanations for these findings is that, when surgeons react angrily to corrective criticism from team members, this reduces the chance that such feedback will be given in the future. This discouragement of criticism can be a conscious or unconscious reason for the angry behaviour and is deleterious for performance. It also seems logical to me that an angry surgeon will be less in control of his actions than a calm one.

A partial answer to this problem can be found in what is called "360 degree feedback". This is a system that is becoming routine in many hospitals, and in which staff and colleagues are expected to monitor each others performance, and give structural honest feedback. Many people are able to self-correct once being made aware of how others see them. This study alone is a powerful argument for the universal implementation of such systems of feedback. One of the best known in the Netherlands is the I.F.M.S. (Individual Functioning Medical Specialist).

A second aspect to the effects of behaviour on performance was highlighted in a study carried out in Florida. During the study there were two groups studied, using infant medical mannequins, in which the doctor was confronted by an actress playing the part of the mother. With a highly critical and argumentative mother, the doctors underperformed on all 11 measures of performance. The effects of the criticism weighed much more heavily than loss of sleep.

The conclusion was that the parental rudeness was affecting the cognitive system negatively, reducing the ability to perform.

There was also some good news: It proved possible, through a computer game using a technique known as cognitive bias modification, to immunise doctors for this effect. If confirmed, it would seem to me that this should become a standard part of all doctor's training, and for that matter, all healthcare workers.

If you can keep your head
when all about you are losing
theirs, it's just possible that
you haven't grasped the
situation

Jean kerr

The empathy spectrum

T he Oxford dictionary defines empathy as the ability to understand and share the feelings of another. The ability to do this depends to some extent on the so called "mirror" neurons in the brain. These neurons can be seen at work when we take on the same posture as someone we feel empathy with. It seems that the ability to feel empathy is at least in part an inherited factor. It is unclear how much we can influence this.

It is probably true that having parents who encourage you to step into the shoes of others, and experience their feelings is relevant for the development of empathy. There is some evidence that it is possible to train empathy in later life. Simply by pretending to be empathic seems to improve this trait, as it brings its own rewards which then can turn pretending into real empathy. This is a parallel with the experiments that demonstrate that by using self-confident body language, you actually develop more self-confidence. "Fake it 'til you make it" is a quote from Amy Cuddy's very enjoyable TED talk "your body language shapes who you are". (Although some other workers have not been able to replicate Cuddy's work, it does seem to me to be incontrovertible that the mind affects our body in many ways, and vice versa)

It is not so that you either do or do not have the ability to feel empathy, it is a spectrum ranging from people who are exquisitely sensitive to other's feelings to people who are completely unable to feel or share them (these are the psychopaths among us). The psychopath may nonetheless be acutely aware of what another is feeling and thinking, and not being encumbered with actually feeling it, they can misuse this knowledge to your detriment. Anyone who finds him or herself near one of these extremes would do well to avoid becoming a doctor. It appears that the psychopathic personality trait is over represented among CEO's. Unfortunately such people do manage to get into medical practice. If they become pathologists or radiologists or take some other function not associated with patient care, then the damage is limited (I am certainly not implying that all radiologists and pathologists are psychopathic, by the way). My brother, who died of cancer a year ago, had the misfortune to have an oncologist who showed no signs of empathy, and if there is one job where empathy is vital, then that's it. As a result of complaints, he is now receiving psychological coaching. I expect the success of this will be limited (see below).

There are two particular difficulties doctors face with regard to empathy. The first is that being too empathic can be the downfall of a doctor. We are faced with so much mental and physical suffering that we have to learn to take some emotional distance, and when confronted with patients we find attractive, we have to put up defensive screens to protect both the patient and ourselves from impossible situations. Another factor is work pressure. During the training and thereafter doctors are in danger of their emotions being blunted by pure tiredness. Finding a balance in all this, in accordance with one's 'inbuilt' empathic qualities is a tricky business. Some doctors may also find that the culture in which they come to work may knock the empathy out of them. It has been said that it is hard to become a surgeon with your empathy intact, as the departmental culture very often just doesn't support it.

A dyslexic child may see his peers reading far better than he can, but cannot understand why. Many such children first draw the conclusion that they must just be stupid. I don't know, but I can imagine a similar reaction when a person with low empathy sees a really good piece of doctor patient interaction. He can probably see that something special is going on, without any internal reference to place it. Result: puzzlement, perhaps frustration.

Although we may be able to learn empathy to some extent, this learning depends on an awareness which is most often absent, and there are surely limits to what can be achieved. A colour blind person will not know he's colour blind if no one tells him. Once a colour blind person realises the nature of the deficit, he cannot learn to see colour; he can learn 'tricks' to

13

help him cope with it — "the top traffic light is red." I would suggest that the same goes for a psychopathic personality. It is important to realise that psychopaths cannot be treated, and that they can be enormously disruptive in a department. In most cases, a good outcome is only possible by removing them.

Take-home message

A healthy amount of empathy is an essential quality for a good doctor. If you've got it, you will know it; if you haven't, then you must hope that someone points it out to you during your training. Then you can decide to do something about it, or make a sensible choice for a specialty with a focus on technique rather than people.

A physician is someone who knows
everything and does nothing.
A surgeon is someone who does
everything and knows nothing.
A psychiatrist is someone who knows
nothing and does nothing
A pathologist is someone who knows
everything and does everything, but a
little too late

Anon

Hold your convictions lightly-

So that you may let them go easily in the light of new evidence.

Having decided what is true, or a fact, or the best option, we have a strong tendency to hold onto those convictions, focus on evidence that supports them, and ignore evidence that negates them. This is called confirmation bias, and is a tendency that can cause serious problems in relationships, and certainly is one of the factors blocking technological progress in the medical world. "We have always done it that way" is often heard. When offered new evidence, there are doctors who are early adopters, and they are the ones who hold their convictions lightly. They are open to, and welcome, the fact that today's truth maybe tomorrow's fallacy, because by being open to this, they are open to new growth. All good qualities suffer when taken to extremes; being too open to new ideas can lead to reckless adoption of new techniques. At the other extreme there are colleagues who hang on tightly to their ideas about how things should be done, and eventually have to be dragged kicking and screaming into a new era.

This resistance to change is partly due to our personalities. When introducing a new computer system to a department, there will be some people who look forward to trying out this new system and discovering what it has to offer. At the other end of the scale there will be people who say, "but it is only 10 years since we had a new system, and it is working fine!" I was known in one hospital where I worked as "Dr Gadget" as a result of the

16

fact that I pounced on any new technology in my eagerness for change. Perhaps this mindset also made it easier for me to accept new ideas and techniques. One example is the 10 years I spent lecturing in and outside of the Netherlands trying to persuade colleagues to use a particular approach for locating and blocking the nerves supplying the arm. I was certain that this was the best and safest approach. Then ultrasound was introduced into regional anaesthesia, and for the first time we could actually visualise the needle and the nerves we wanted to anaesthetise. Suddenly the arguments I had used for my technique lost much of their validity. Fortunately I held my convictions lightly enough that I was able to let go, and switch to the use of ultrasound and an alternative technique. Since then, ultrasound guided nerve block has become the new standard, and there is little doubt that it is safer, more effective and less unpleasant for the patient. And yet I know of one highly prominent professor of anaesthesia who for many years, and despite all the evidence to the contrary, still refused to use ultrasound or admit to its advantages. He was unable to let go of the convictions he held so tightly. It must have cost a lot of energy simply trying to defend the indefensible until reality set in, and he embraced the new technique.

Apart from having a personality that is uniquely for or against change, there is another reason why people find it hard to change their opinions; if they change their mind, then they believe they have previously been "wrong". Admitting this is difficult for many, and has much to do with culture, upbringing, and of course the ego (see the chapter on cognitive dissonance).

Take home message

Changing your mind can be a sign of growth.

If you are distressed by anything external, the pain is not due to the thing itself, but your estimate of it; and this you have the power to revoke at any moment

Marcus Aurelius

Just be yourself

I t sounds so obvious, doesn't it? Why would one not want to be one-self? But it's not that easy, especially for a young doctor. It is a question of egos again: what makes it hard is that we are often not all that satisfied with ourselves. We look at all the self-confident colleagues around us and think it better not to show our uncertainties, or ignorance or doubts about our competence too clearly. What is often missed is the truth that that is exactly what most of those "self-confident" colleagues are also going through. They have just learned to wear a mask.

The herd instinct is also powerful. If you join a team in which it is considered normal to treat juniors or lower graded staff with disdain, it is much easier to make this approach your own. Attempts to treat members inside and outside the department with respect and as equals will be seen as weakness by some colleagues, and if you persist, and become more liked than they are, you may also be confronted with jealousy. This is how a departmental culture is created and perpetuated. People with low self-esteem tend to give way to these pressures. People with high self-esteem will find it easier to ignore such duress, and just be themselves.

Our susceptibility to social pressures goes far further than most people realise. One extraordinary example of this was the social experiment carried out by Derren Brown, and filmed for a television programme called "The Push" in which he looked to see whether he could use social pressures to get someone to commit murder in the space of a couple of hours. It's a fascinating piece of television, can be seen on Netflix and probably You-Tube, and I shall give no spoilers.

Low self-esteem is unfortunately pervasive in our culture. If you were lucky then you will have had parents who were able to give you unconditional love; you grew up with the feeling that you are "o.k." without having to do anything to earn that feeling. Unfortunately this is more the exception than the rule. Most of us learn that we are conditionally o.k. We are o.k. when we come up to the expectations of our "elders and betters" or social group. Before we blame our parents for this it is good to realise that this is a multi-generational thing. Our parents could not give to us what they had not received themselves. Only once we are aware of this do we have a chance to break the chain and give our children a better start in life. Even this is not easy if your own self-esteem is less than optimal; if we manage to make it a little easier for each successive generation then we may be satisfied.

Unfortunately the price for not daring to be our-self is high. By not admitting that we do not know something, we miss the chance to learn, and because we treat patients on the basis of our knowledge, we do them a poor service when we have to guess at what we do not know. We also then live under heightened tension as we always have the fear of being found out. I remember well how I was when I first started giving lessons to anaesthetic trainees. I felt that I should be able to answer all their questions, and felt warm under the collar when I could not. I tried talking round the subject hoping they would not penetrate my ignorance (they did). I can't tell you what a relief it was when I learned to say, "I've no idea! Look it up and tell me about it next lesson". What a weight fell off my shoulders! And I'm certain that my students liked and respected me the better for daring to be vulnerable, as we set out on a path of learning together.

(I don't know that admitting to ignorance is always the best course. In my own job, I had on average about 7 minutes to prepare a new patient for an anaesthetic. In that time I had to create a feeling of trust, discuss past history, treatment choices and other relevant medical issues. Then it all had to be written down or entered in the computer. You can imagine that there was little time for small talk. Patients have high expectations of your competence and knowledge. In the last years, I always had my computer logged in to Google. If someone came in with a some unusual syndrome, and I had never heard of it, admitting to this would give me another 6 minutes to regain their dented confidence. So I'm afraid that I resorted to a little sub-terfuge: I would say, "ah! Grobbly's syndrome, let me just check the latest information on that". Well, it wasn't totally dishonest, and they probably left the room with more trust than otherwise would have been the case (and perhaps more than I deserved)! I am a great believer in being open with my patients, but as with so many things, being absolute in such matters is sometimes kinder to one's own conscience than to the patient.)

Let me give you a clearer example of someone going to great lengths to cover his ignorance and technical shortcomings: I worked for a number of years with a colleague anaesthetist who had managed to scrape through his training with virtually no experience of regional anaesthesia techniques (anaesthetising an arm or a leg, or the lower half of the body are examples). He was an ill fit in our club, because we were highly oriented to these tech-niques. His approach was to claim that regional techniques were unneces-sary and even dangerous. He went so far as to warn a patient who had re-quested epidural anaesthesia for a cesarean section that it could kill her. He often had to be helped out by his own assistants when he couldn't manage a spinal anaesthetic. He made a bit of a laughing stock of himself, and of course suffered a great deal of stress. He developed high blood pressure and was eventually put out to graze. This drama could have had a positive ending if only he had dared to be himself. He could simply have said, "I'm not good at these things — will you help me learn?" Or "can we arrange that I do the general anaesthetics, you the regional anaesthesia?" He would have gained respect, and would certainly have received the support of his colleagues. I presume that his self-esteem was so low that he feared that if he were to be open he would be laughed at. If only he had known!

Dr. Peter Reid was Head of the Anaesthetic department in Canterbury, England, where I did my training for my fellowship. I was the most junior in the department and was surprised when a nurse came to me to ask me if I would help Dr Reid out with a problem with a patient in the operating room. It was solved easily enough, because the answer lay in the theory I was just studying. My admiration for him has always remained with me, not because the rookie in the department was able to help the chief, but because the chief was able to be so vulnerable that he asked the rookie to come and help him. This is now teaching by example!

I remember when I was just qualified as a doctor in St. Andrews in Scotland. I was driving my family just after my graduation ceremony when we witnessed a car accident. The ambulance was just arriving. I looked at the victim and pronounced her dead. A lady standing next to me said that she had a first aid diploma and that the patient was still alive! You can bet that I followed that ambulance to the hospital and was somewhat relieved (!!!) to see her confirmed dead. What a terrible admission! But it does show how very inadequate and uncertain I felt; I was a doctor, but what did I really know when it came to the crunch?

Shortly after that I was doing my first weeks as an intern on a surgical ward. A patient complained of headache, and I told the Staff nurse to give him an aspirin. "The patient does have a gastric ulcer, doctor," she replied. Oops! Not a good idea to give aspirin to someone with a stomach ulcer. I can't remember how I reacted. I hope I was able to say, "Thank you so much nurse, I have much to learn." I rather fear, however, that I just turned red and muttered something under my breath. I was not very good at the vulnerability thing back then!

I am now retired, and doing locum work because I enjoy spending time with patients and colleagues. At present I am in the fortunate position to be supervising trainee anaesthetists. I try to make sure that Dr Reid's lesson is not lost. The juniors are much more up-to-date than I am. With time one loses a lot of knowledge which becomes compensated for by experience. So the juniors bring me back up to date and I share with them what the years have taught me.

People who dare to be vulnerable are the people we can have a warm and open contact with. People who hide their vulnerability behind a screen of confidence are the people we never quite seem to know. The screen hides more than their weaknesses.

Take-home message:

I suppose the lesson to be learned from all this is that we have our strong and our weak points, and that we can best improve the weak points by being open and vulnerable, and being prepared to learn from everyone around us. A counter argument is that being vulnerable is just that — that there will be people who will use your openness and honesty against you. There are such people, and they can be a pain in the neck. But for each of these there will be ten who will like and respect you more for your courage to show your vulnerable side. Someone who can say, "I don't know," or "I am not good at that," is someone who will learn quicker and be a better doctor in the long term.

Advice is what we ask for when we already know the answer, but with we didn't

Erica Jong

Seek first to understand

and then to be understood

I f I was asked to give one take-home message to anyone in any situation where communication is needed, it would be this chapter heading, which I found in the brilliant book, "The Seven Habits of Highly Effective People" by Stephen Covey. To my mind nothing is more powerful in improving communication and relationships, and probably nothing more simple (which, by the way, is not quite the same as easy).

I have my own ideas about things and my own way of doing them. I am aware that there are other ideas and other ways of doing things, but I think and do it my way because I think it is "better" or "right". By extension, your ideas and ways of doing things, if different, are worse, or wrong. So when we sit opposite each other in an argument I don't want to waste too much time listening to your wrong ideas — why would I? While you are talking I am busy planning how to dismantle your arguments and cannot wait to start persuading you to change your mind. So you are talking, and I am not listening.

The map is not the territory

"The map is not the territory" is a statement attributed to Gregory Bateson, English anthropologist, social scientist, linguist, visual anthropologist, semiotician, and cyberneticist, and points to a very important distinction. I shall try to make it clear. If I want to travel by car from Antwerp to Liege in

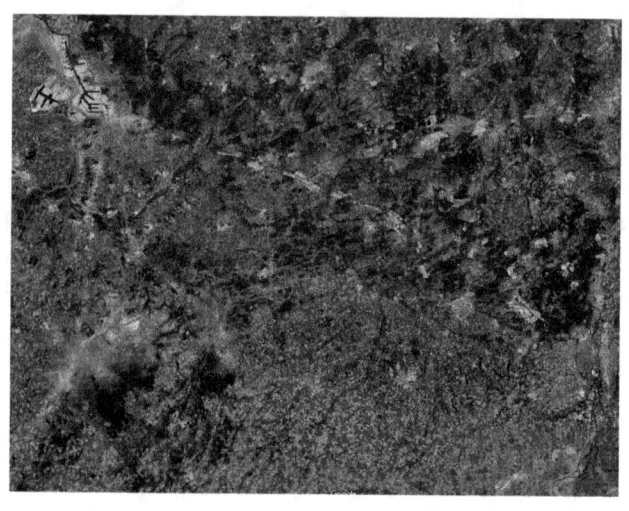

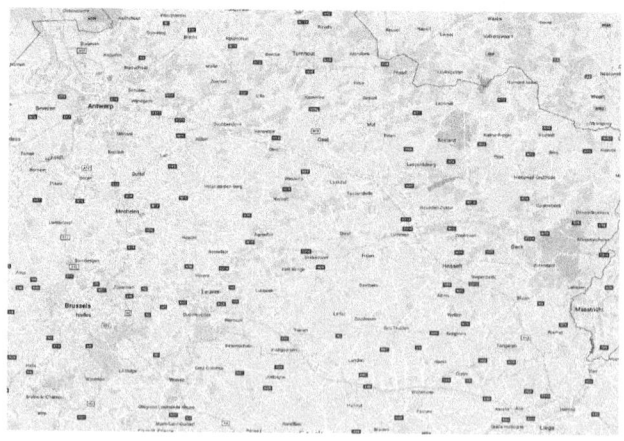

Belgium, I could open Google maps in satellite view. This would be at the same time a very accurate map, and completely useless. It contains far too

much information, 99% of which is not relevant to what I want to do. Google understands this and therefore makes a simplified map which only shows the roads and built-up areas. This map is useful and accurate for achieving our aims. But of course, if we wanted to do the same journey by boat, we should need an entirely different map, with canals and rivers. This could then also be accurate and sufficient to achieve our aim. It is however a totally different map, and neither are an accurate representation of the territory between these two cities. So the map is not the territory.

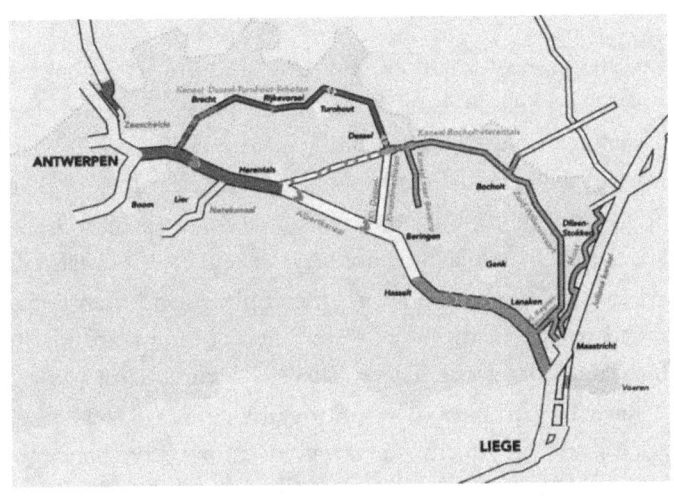

The same thing goes on in our minds: we are simply not capable of registering or coping with all the details of the world about us. We filter 99% out, and make a map of the world in our heads which is certainly not accurate, but hopefully sufficient to achieve our ends. Everybody does the same, so that life is full of different maps and different aims. That does not need to be a problem; all these maps can enrich one another. For this enrichment, one condition must be met, and that is that we respect the maps others have. This is unfortunately the exception; usually we assume that our map is the correct one, and thus that the other has it wrong. And of course, sometimes they do have it wrong, and sometimes we do.

If you believe in a God, it may be that your mind has a map in which religion is seen as a plain with a high mountain representing the positive aspects, and a small dip beneath sea level representing the negative aspects. As an atheist, in my world map, it is the opposite, with a deep ocean representing the negative aspects of religion, and a small island with a palm tree to represent the positive. Among people who agree that there is a God, you will find the next level of maps. The Christian has a different map to a radical Islamist. Among Christians, you will see the next level, with different maps for a moderate Christian and an Evangelical Christian. This is why discussions on religion (or politics, for that matter) are often so fruitless and heated. It's about, "Your map is wrong, and I shall prove it to you," and this is behind the advice to avoid discussing these subjects in "polite company".

Let us come back to the case of my colleague from the previous chapter who was not competent in regional anaesthesia. It was three of us and one of him. We stated our position, he stated his. We were right and he was wrong; that was clear (to us then)! It was probably just as clear to him that we were wrong and he was being bullied. It was a classical example of a conflict between specialists in which positions are taken on the basis of information we have available (which is always incomplete), and then these positions are defended to the death, as it were. Such conflicts are rarely solved to the satisfaction of all parties. There is usually a winner and a loser. And if the parties have to continue working together, there is really no winner — the "loser" is now an "enemy," and will look for every chance to even up the score.

The only way to come to a satisfactory solution is to get past the positions and down to the underlying motives and emotions. It has been said, "Solve the emotions and the problem often evaporates" And I know from experience how true this is. The great Sufi poet Rumi said it beautifully: "Out beyond ideas of wrong-doing and right-doing there is a field. I will meet you there."

The correct approach is very simple; just listen and ask background questions until you have thoroughly understood where the other is coming from. The reward for your patience is twofold and great. In the first place the other may come up with ideas that you've never thought of and, God forbid, you might even just come to the conclusion that he is right! End of conflict (at least, if you have the courage to admit that). If that is not the

28

case you have still done something powerful; you have shown the other that you are interested in his or her ideas. I cannot over-emphasise how important people find it to have someone listen to them, to be heard. The likelihood that they will then be prepared to listen to you will be enormously increased. The fact that you have shown interest in, and listened to each other makes the likelihood of a solution that satisfies both far greater.

This listening has to be done with genuine interest and respect. Being honestly curious about others is a tremendously powerful instrument in helping them to open up to you. And it works to the advantage of both parties. Instead of having created a loser, an enemy as it were, you have laid the foundations for a productive working relationship. In the process of listening to each other you will unavoidably see the other in a more positive light simply because you know him or her better.

On very many occasions the other will tell you something which stops you dead in your tracks, and makes you say, "I'm sorry, I never knew that." For instance, if I had engaged in this sort of conversation with my colleague I might have learned that he had a patient who had a serious nerve injury after a spinal anaesthetic he had performed, and that this was very traumatic for him. In that case I would undoubtedly have been much more understanding, and maybe we would have come to a better understanding.

As I read this back, it all seems so obvious. It may seem superfluous to write it all down. However the truth is that, however obvious, it is not the way it usually happens: then it is business as usual, taking in positions and defending them with scant regard for what is playing in the mind of the other. Admitting that the other is right implies that we are wrong, and our delicate egos will go a long way to avoid that conclusion.

Take home message

Be aware that this pattern of taking and defending positions and of wanting to be right is deeply ingrained in most of us, that it is generally destructive and that the rewards for changing this pattern are great.

N.B. I stand by this chapter, and believe that it is one of the most valuable pieces of advice I can pass on. But honesty obliges me to say that while this is true for the vast majority of relationships, there are still people who are mentally so disturbed, or with such fragile egos, that the formation of a partnership of trust and mutual respect is just not going to be possible; in which the only way to work together seems to be to flatter them, and to submit to their will. It is true for psychopaths and malignant narcissists, for instance, who are far more numerous in important positions that many would think possible. They can be particularly adept at knowing how others are feeling and thinking, without the encumbrance of feeling any shame or remorse. There can come a time when, in order to protect one's own integrity, it is better to simply avoid such people where possible. Alas, I have worked with some such, and learned that flattery and subservience are no answer in the long term.

I am writing this book at a time when Donald Trump is president of the United States. When I see how he taints all who work with him, how they almost all leave under a black cloud when he discovers there are limits to their loyalty and obedience, then it remains incredible that there are still people prepared of their own free will to go and work for him. I can only think of blind ambition, or an equally blind and naive loyalty to a greater cause. If you are not convinced that flattery and subservience will be your own undoing, I suggest studying American political life in 2018; it is full of public figures who will be consigned to the trash heap of history. Remaining true to yourself can be difficult, but your integrity is too valuable to give away.

I don't want to achieve immortality through my work. I want to achieve it through not dying.

Woody Allen

Please take your hat off

I understand that airline pilots are no longer allowed to wear their hats in the cockpit because these can be a symbol of dominance and power. The Busby is another fine example; the royal guards look taller and more fearsome. We are wired-in to look up with respect to tall people; it is no coincidence that the taller of the two candidates almost always wins in United States Presidential elections.

This business of hats in the cockpit has its roots in a terrible accident between two Boeing 747 aircraft on the island of Tenerife in 1977 in which 583 people died. As in most aircraft accidents, this one was caused by a number of factors: a bomb scare on Gran Canaria airport, causing a number of planes to be diverted to the small Los Rodeos airport which was physically not well equipped to take many large aircraft. The taxiway was blocked by parked aircraft, and communications between the tower and the two aircraft involved were not optimal. At the time of the accident, the airport was covered in clouds with very low visibility, and the two jumbo jets involved had to taxi out on the main runway to position themselves for take-off. However the direct cause of the accident was a bad decision by the KLM captain.

He was a man with more than 11,000 hours of flying experience. He was apparently stressed and irritable, and was determined to take off as soon as possible (for quite understandable reasons). He started to take off without proper clearance from the control tower, and ignored comments from his crew suggesting that another 747 might still be on the runway. The KLM aircraft took off, saw the Pan Am aircraft too late, and ploughed into it. This incident was one of the wake-up calls for the development of Crew Resource Management (CRM), and one the chief aims was to level out the power structure. It was very difficult for his crew to question a decision taken by somebody of such vast experience and seniority.

Reportedly, KLM wanted to get their chief flying officer to investigate the causes of the accident, but discovered that he was the one who had caused it! So no matter how senior, how experienced and highly skilled, we can all make mistakes, and we all need to be able to accept criticism from juniors.

Of course there are limits to this — in general the captain's decisions should be better than those of the co-pilot, as is dictated by experience and training. But he will have his blind spots, and will sometimes be over-tired or occupied by private problems. And then it is essential that the threshold be as low as possible for input from the junior. In times of split-second judgement, the captain has to use his authority; at other times he would do well to use the collective wisdom of his crew.

This is highly relevant for hospital practice, and when things goes wrong it also costs lives. It is true that my younger son, who is a pilot, can kill hundreds at one time, whereas I can only do it one by one, but the lesson is clear. For this reason many hospitals are introducing CRM training for medical staff.

What does this mean for the doctor? It means that the junior needs to be assertive, and if he or she is not that by nature, then an assertiveness training would be good for the doctor, and perhaps life-saving for the patient. Most of us get little training in assertiveness, and one of the most common alternatives is to react with passive aggression. A good example of this was when a surgeon was coping with major blood-loss during an abdominal operation. The anaesthetist, instead of mentioning his concerns in an assertive manner, said, "Shall I hang up another bag of blood, or shall I pour it straight into the abdomen?" This was not the start of a constructive exchange!

For the senior doctor, awareness of this problem is vital, and the fact that he or she is not above criticism should be made clear to their juniors, and they should be thankful when important feedback is given. In practice it is my experience that many specialists are insecure and probably fear that accepting criticism is a slippery slope on which their dominant position may be in for a fall. We are back to the ego. They are also aware at some, often repressed, level that there are so many things in their job that they perhaps should know, but do not. One small example to demonstrate this is when the specialist is asked by an assistant how much of a drug to inject. I have heard on occasion the reaction "give one ampoule," which neatly disguises the fact that he does not know the dose, but does know that the contents of an ampoule are usually safe to inject. This sounds terrible, but it is not rare. Opening up to criticism might demonstrate some of these blind spots. Funnily enough, for all their concern for their ego, doctors who do not cope well with feedback, end up not liked and not respected.

Take home message

It is an unfortunate fact that for many, respect is not something we have to earn — for them it goes with the hat. The lessons learned from air accidents are very clearly applicable to the hospital situation, and implementation of Crew Resource Management will lead to increased safety, and a more healthy and happy working climate. The advantages apply just as much for the ones at the top of the ladder and it is a pity that they often show the most resistance to such change, which superficially seems to threaten them, but actually supports and strengthens their position.

> Do or do not
> There is no try

Yoda

Should we really want to emulate the

pilots?

For many years the behavioural codes and training of pilots (Crew Resource Management) has been held up as an example which should be followed in health services, especially on departments such as the operating theatres, intensive care and traumatology. Many specialists look on this as a trendy fad, and relatively little effort is put into implementing changes to follow the example. How necessary is it? As you read the following about the airline industry, I would ask you to look for parallels with the hospital experience.

The basic assumption is, that if an accident has happened once, the chances are that it will happen again sometime in the future, unless steps are taken to prevent this. This is why in the air transportation industry enormous amounts of time, money and energy are spent in analysing each accident. The results of the investigations are made known worldwide, and recommendations are given as to how it may be avoided in the future. This may be in the form of design changes, cultural changes, training improvements or improved operational procedures.

The changes implemented in the design of aircraft, training of crew and operational procedures have led to a vast improvement in safety. This procedure is one of the main reasons that flying has become the safest form of transport.

In almost every situation it is found that a number of factors add up together before an accident happens. This has been described as the Swiss cheese model. The cheese is full of holes, and the chance that all of these holes will line up is very small, but also clearly possible.

The diagrams below demonstrate a situation in which a patient gets an allergic reaction and while the team is dealing with this, a ventilator dysfunction occurs. The oximeter, which measures oxygen in the blood, warns of impending problems, and a serious incident is avoided. In the second case the team forget to attach the oximeter to the patient, and on instructions of the surgeon, they inject a dye, which turns the patient blue. Because the anaesthetic team expects the patient to turn blue, they are not alarmed by the colour. This series of events can lead to them losing the patient. Each problem on its own would not have led to a serious incident and this lulls us into a sense of false security.

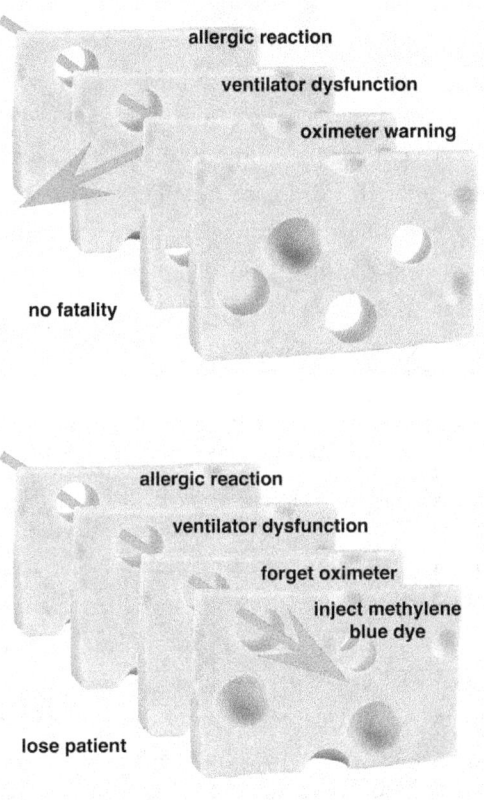

However unlikely, the coincidence of them all happening at the same time will happen sometime, somewhere (just like the four old ladies playing a game of bridge who discovered that each of them had been dealt a full suite of cards, or the idea that if you put a number of monkeys behind typewriters, given sufficient time they would eventually type the complete works of Shakespeare purely by chance).

We have already discussed the question of authority in the previous chapter. There is still a large step between saying that the captain is not above criticism, and this actually being the case in the cockpit or at the operating table.

It demands a change in culture, which only really happens once the person in the position of authority becomes aware of his own fallibility, and that being challenged may be vitally important to him personally, and not just seen as a loss of authority.

Crew resource management goes further than this. It also involves analysing how a team works together, and communicates together. It implies that each crew member needs to be aware of his own strong and weak points, and those of his colleagues. It involves learning to communicate unequivocally and without blaming. The captain will not say, for instance, "It's your turn now," or, "can I hand over to you now?" He will simply say, "Controls are yours". And his co-pilot will confirm with "my controls". Using a very clear set of standardised phrases means that even in stress situations, the chances of misunderstanding are reduced to a minimum, and it is clear for every crew member what is expected from him or her. This just does not happen in the great majority of operating theatres. There is no standardised vocabulary, and there is rarely verbal confirmation. I am perfectly certain that this leads to many unnecessary mistakes and deaths.

In the cockpit of an aircraft, in order to maximise the chance of avoiding problems, and to deal efficiently with them when they do crop up, a whole complicated series of standard operating procedures has been developed. Standard operating procedures (SOP), have great advantages, but there is also the downside, and that is that it reduces initiative and flexibility in the pilots. In 2009, US airways Flight 1549, which lost power to both engines and was safely landed on the Hudson River with no loss of life, was an example of "thinking out of the box". There was no protocol to save these lives, just the captain's experience and courage to follow his own instincts. The fascinating film documentary "Sully" describes how the pilot was initially criticised for not following the SOP, and how he was eventually vindicated. Rigidly applying protocols can limit the application and development of original solutions. Airlines are coming back to some extent on a very rigid set of operating procedures to take account of this. A middle of the road approach is best, and this also applies in hospitals, where protocols can sometimes cause more problems than they solve.

Adhering blindly to complicated protocols sometimes leads to enormous and unnecessary expense, and to a sort of blindness. A good example of this was all of the preoperative investigations that we used to carry out. In the 1980s every patient over the age of 40 years had a battery of blood tests done, an electrocardiogram and a chest x-ray. They were also often sent routinely to the physician for a medical check. Research in America showed that to find one abnormality that would lead to the death of the patient would cost millions of dollars. What was even worse, was that they discovered that because the chance of finding a relevant abnormality was so very low, abnormal findings were very often overlooked. I write deliberately "relevant" because many abnormalities would turn up, but they were usually not relevant for whether an anaesthetic could be given safely. So after spending those millions of dollars, the one significant result which you needed to save your patient's life got snowed under in the avalanche of data. These days, preoperative investigations are largely done when there is a specific indication. This reduces the cost enormously, and makes it far more likely that abnormal findings will be noticed. It may be imagined that the radiologists and physicians were not uniformly enthusiastic about these changes as it led to a significant reduction in referrals and x-rays and blood tests, which had a considerable effect on their earnings. In my small hospital alone, the number of chest x-rays was reduced from hundreds per year to almost zero with the patients being no worse off.

It is important to distinguish here the difference between a general population screening and a preoperative screening. With a greatly reduced number of investigations we shall certainly miss some unexpected diagnoses, such as a lung tumour on the chest x-ray. However if screening for lung cancer is considered valuable, it should be carried out on the whole population, and not be seen as a by-product of pre-operative screening in a sub-population. When done as a means to it's own end — i.e. diagnosing cancer in an early stage, then abnormalities will be better noticed, as they are not just turning up in a mass of largely irrelevant information. That said, the value of mass screening programmes is not always what one might expect. They can also lead to over-diagnosis and over-treatment.

Crew resource management also concerns itself with what is called situational awareness. When we are highly concentrated on a particular problem, we tend to lose sight of what is happening around us. In this way one aircraft crash (Eastern Air Lines Flight 401) was caused because the pilots were so concerned about a warning light on the undercarriage control that they failed to notice that they were running out of fuel. The worst of it was that there was no actual problem with the undercarriage, and simply a false alarm. There were 101 fatalities. Situational awareness is vitally important, as is dividing the work among crew members to ensure that all aspects are covered, even when one particular problem is demanding a high degree of concentration.

Situational awareness is just as big of an issue in the operating theatre. In one well publicised case, a young woman was undergoing anaesthesia that required that a tube be put into her airway. This proved unexpectedly difficult, and the whole anaesthetic team was so focussed on getting the tube in place, that they lost all sense of time, and even ignored a theatre nurse who had fetched an emergency tracheotomy set, which would have saved the patient's life. The patient died of lack of oxygen.

Another important part of crew resource management is the briefing and debriefing. During the briefing the crew discuss the important points in the upcoming flight, and try to flag potential problems. During the debriefing, the flight is reviewed, and crew members are expected to point out any problem situations that occurred, and when there has been an accident or a mistake made, to report this. The whole point of the debriefing is that it is seen as a moment to learn and improve safety. Absolutely essential in this procedure is that crew members feel safe to report any mistakes which they have made themselves. It is about what went wrong, and not who did wrong. If crew members are not certain of this and feel in anyway unsafe reporting mistakes, then they will simply not report which also means that mistakes cannot be learned from.

In my opinion, all of the above points can be so clearly translated to the hospital environment that it seems unthinkable that we do not apply what has been learned in the airline industry to our own work. However, when we look at operating theatres and intensive care departments, we find very few of the protective measures which have made flying so much safer.

In the past few years at least a briefing has been introduced in the form of a timeout procedure immediately before an operation is carried out. This may be compared to the pilot's pre-flight briefing, and has been demonstrated to reduce the number of medical missers (such as operations on the wrong side). In the past years we have also seen an increase in the number of protocols for the different procedures used in the department. Nonetheless I have seen many surgeons trying to avoid or undermine the timeout procedure at any cost and this is quite inexplicable to me. Unfortunately this timeout is about the only way that I have seen the lessons from crew resource management being translated to the operating theatre. A debriefing after the operation is pretty rare. An open and non-blaming atmosphere so that mistakes are reported freely is in my experience more the exception than the rule. I have seen on so many occasions a surgeon getting in trouble and doing his best to shift the blame onto his assistants or onto the anaesthetic team. There is almost no structure for the systematic reporting of unwanted events to colleagues worldwide. A few medical societies have introduced a system in which information over quality improvements and accidents is shared, and this has proven to be very successful. But it is a long way from being universal.

One reason why it is taking so long to introduce these practices is that there is at the time of writing an increasing pressure to cut costs. The implementation of safe practices costs time, and that implies either more efficient working methods, or more staff to carry out the extra work. Up to a point, efficiency may be improved by more intelligent use of personnel and technology, but in my experience it often simply comes down to getting more work out of the same number of people which leads eventually to more stress, demotivation and increased sick leave. Then these workers are expected to introduce Crew Resource Management and it is hardly surprising that it happens half-heartedly.

One other reason why the pressure to introduce these methods was much greater in the airline industry is that when an aircraft crashes we often talk about hundreds of deaths of healthy people, and it is worldwide news. When something goes wrong in the operating theatres it involves usually just one person, and in many cases they are ill before the operation begins. It is so much easier to sweep these instances under the carpet, something quite unthinkable when an aircraft crashes.

In some situations, crew resource management has been applied systematically to a department. This was the case in the intensive care department of the Radboud University Medical Centre in Nijmegen in the Netherlands. After the introduction of these procedures, the number of cardiac arrests was drastically reduced, and the success rate of resuscitation improved considerably.

Since writing the first draft of this book I am glad to report that at least one hospital, the Radboud University Medical Centre is seriously applying CRM principles on the Operating theatres. The experience is highly positive, and where I feared that it would not be taken up because of the extra time needed for the procedure, it turns out that time is actually won due to increased efficiency, and reduction in cancellation of operations.

Take-home message

Yes, we really should want to emulate the pilots. Crew resource management, similar to that carried out in the airline industry, should be introduced to every operating theatre, intensive care and emergency department. Much effort will need to be applied to create cultural changes so that workers in these departments welcome crew resource management instead of seeing it as another bureaucratic way of spilling their valuable time.

Patients who are asked, "Is there *something* else?" will much more often raise other considerations than when asked, "is there *anything* else?"

Word choice matters!

National Ambulatory Medical Care Survey

There is no failure

— only feedback

The heading of this chapter is a pre-supposition, and as with all of these, it is not so much an absolute truth as it is a pragmatic approach to life. The medical world is reasonably competitive, and a polarisation into success and failure is not unusual. The trouble with viewing actions as failures is that it tends to put us into a negative mental frame, and a downward spiral. If you see the result as feedback, then it is also a moment to learn and grow. That is what this presupposition is about. The example of feedback most often quoted is Edison, who tried many times without success to make a practical light bulb. Edison became famous for saying, "I have not failed 10,000 times. I have not failed once. I have succeeded in proving that those 10,000 ways will not work. When I have eliminated the ways that will not work, I will find the way that will work." And he did.

This is a mental choice: am I going to see this as a series of failures (depressing and demotivating) or as a pathway to success (empowering)? This may sound like splitting hairs, but it is one reason why some people give up easily when confronted with obstacles, and others push ahead to success. We have a choice.

It is also good to accept that 'failure' is an essential part of learning. You can't learn to walk without falling over, you can't learn to play tennis without hitting the ball out many times and indeed there is no activity that you can learn to do well without going through the learning curve, and that means that at first you will not do it well — there will be "failures". So the important lesson to learn is the mental trick of turning "I have failed" into "I am learning and growing".

The mental dissonance caused by the combined mindset of, "I have failed" with "I must not make mistakes" is the cause of a very familiar pattern — that of "other blaming". Some specialists seem to think that that is what nurses and assistants are for — to take the blame. I always say (as a joke, honest!) that if anything goes wrong, the nurse gets the blame first and when they refuse to accept it, the patient is next in line; only in very extreme cases will I take the blame myself. Unfortunately this happens (probably daily) in every hospital I have worked in. And if I am really honest, then I am no doubt guilty of it myself from time to time. And we don't really get away with it, because it is often visible to everyone except the blamer.

Some of my surgical colleagues are especially adept at this, and probably have more targets than most. When the operation is not going well, the anaesthetist can be blamed for not providing enough muscle relaxation, the assistant for not holding the instruments properly, the circulating nurse for not aiming the light into the wound. In my experience it is unusual for a surgeon to say, "I'm stuck, would you ask Dr. A if he would come and help me?" More common is that the scrub nurse says (usually very carefully), "Would it be an idea to ask Dr. A to come and help?" "No, it would not" is the usual answer.

Take home message

Accept that you are not perfect, that you will make mistakes, and be comfortable with that. When you make a mistake, don't beat yourself up about it. Look at it with curiosity instead of anger to see how it came about, and how you may learn from it. I can guarantee you that you will feel happier, and that your performance will improve quicker if you follow this approach.

My parents have been visiting me for a few days.
I just dropped them off at the airport.
They leave tomorrow.

Margaret Smith

Try to catch people out doing things well

I have made a habit of giving compliments dating from my time as a medical student in St. Andrews university in Scotland. I lived in student accommodation where our meals were prepared in a central kitchen and consumed in a communal dining room. I noticed how the other students were quick to complain when the food was not good, and said nothing when it *was* good. I decided to do the opposite, and to make a long story short, when it was cherry cream pie day, I always got a second portion (and the third was hidden away for me under the stairs).

What I have never understood is why it is that people in general are so quick to criticise and so slow to compliment when there is every reason to do the opposite. Negative criticism pulls people down, demotivates them, makes them dislike you, makes them uncertain and perform at a lower level. Who in their right mind would want to achieve these things?

My wife came home the other day with a story about a young assistant, who was being introduced to the task of taking blood samples from patients. After a week she was to be evaluated to see if she could continue in the job. The first day my wife worked with her, and the assistant took her blood samples with success with each patient. The following day she was with a hyper-critical colleague who was more interested in demonstrating her own abilities. At the end of the day the poor girl was so unsure of herself, that the next day she refused to take blood samples. At the end of the week it was my wife's task to undo the damage done by her colleague. I'm sure there was no deliberate attempt to undermine her sense of competence, it was just that the ego of the supervisor got in the way, and the supervisor was probably totally unaware that young people tend to live up (or down) to expectations.

I think that the metaphor of the emotional bank account is an especially powerful one. This metaphor is relevant whether it concerns parents and children, colleagues or doctors with their assistants. See criticism as making a withdrawal, and complimenting as making a deposit. Some people are chronically "in the red".

As an example I can take the holding area of the large hospital where I am currently working. I want my operating programmes to run efficiently and I am heavily dependent on the nursing staff working there. They can make or break my day. At the time of writing I have had a very busy day, and thanks to the nursing staff and my assistants it ran like clockwork. At the end of the day I expressed my appreciation in a note I stuck on their notice board. This had never happened before and was a very significant deposit in the emotional bank account. This means two things; next time I am doubly assured of them going the extra mile for me. When I am dissatisfied, I can express this with less resistance because I have built up credit. It is also a way to create a team who enjoy working together. It has, to my mind, no downside. This very simple approach makes both sides happier and more effective.

There are colleagues who do the opposite; needless to say they are constantly overdrawn and the nurses will do the bare minimum to help them. This increases the negative comments of the doctor and nobody is happy at the end of the day.

There is nothing holy in this approach. It is a truly win-win way of interacting with others.

Take home message

If you focus on what is positive in other people's behaviour you will help them to improve their performance and self-esteem, and *you* will be one of the main beneficiaries.

Fear is the main cause of superstition, and one of the main sources of cruelty, to conquer fear is the beginning of wisdom

Bertrand Russel

What's in a name?

When I was about fourteen years old I bought a book by Harry Lo-rayne on memory techniques. One sentence has always stuck in my mind: "a person's name is their most valuable possession". More on names in a moment; first I should like to write a little on memory.

In the same book the author points out that many people say that their memory is like a sieve, and that every time we write something down to remember it, we make another hole in the sieve, and every time we entrust it to memory, we close a hole. Well put, I think. Memory systems have been around for thousands of years. A Roman general knew the names of all the soldiers in his army. Simonides came up with a system in 477BC. After a building collapsed where a feast was being given he was able to name all the guests and knew who had sat where. Most modern methods are based on his system of loci. And they work, and they can be amazingly efficient.

My 'inbuilt' memory is no better or worse than that of anyone else and yet using that system I was able to memorise the entire London underground system; I could give all the stations in the right order, and where you should change lines to get somewhere. At that time it had about 150 stations and about ten different lines. It was not entirely practical as I rarely used the underground, but it was a good exercise! I also learned all the 250 or so telephone numbers in my hospital in Winterswijk, including those in the lifts, just to be complete. What do you mean neurotic? More useful was learning the week's operating schedules by heart. I had so often met patients in the corridors and thought, "Who is that?" After memorising them, I recognised them all, knew who had operated on them and why and how old they were. "So where's the catch?" you may ask. Well, the catch is that it requires time and discipline, and both are often in short supply. The frustrating thing is that I am sure that if I had spent some more time actively using it, then it would have become quick, automatic and unconscious — thus taking neither time nor discipline. I shall always regret not getting that far.

Back to names. I do believe that names are important. If someone uses our first name, it is like a warm touch. But names are tricky. To start with, when someone introduces themselves, we often don't even register the name properly. If we do, it goes into the short term memory, and by the time we say good bye, we've lost it already. And certainly in the hospital world, we walk into a new job, and get introduced to dozens of people, one after another. In my experience, by the time I have heard the third name, I've forgotten the other two. The second thing that makes it tricky, at least in my case, is that, after I have been working with people for a month or so, I am ashamed to ask them again. I am not proud of it, but after twelve years of working in one hospital, I slunk past some of the receptionists every day, not knowing their names.

It doesn't have to be that way, and there are a few general tips you can use. The first is, repeat the name back to them, and if there is anything unusual about it, ask. This ensures that the name has at least entered you short-term memory. Then it is valuable to use the name a few times in the first conversation, to start getting it moving to the medium term memory. Not too much — you will get queer looks! After that use it every time you meet them, and if you forget, ask again. People won't mind you doing this; it's a compliment.

For doctors and nurses, it is important to remember the names of their patients. It can be quite a challenge. There are days when you have fifteen people to treat in the operating theatre. It is busy, you get tired. Before you know it you are talking about "this patient," or "Mr. Umm...er...". I worked in one hospital where one of the anaesthetic assistants always knew the names of his patients, and used these names to address them. I have tried to learn from him. In the Netherlands it is even easier to go wrong than in English, as it is in general use to say "mister" or "misses" without adding the surname when talking to patients. I know for certain that patients appreciate hearing their names instead.

Of course it is possible to learn and use a memory system, as I did in the past, but I fear that it is too much of a bother for most people.

I have a system of my own which works well, but takes effort (as does everything that is worth-while). When I started working in a large hospital in Rotterdam I was confronted with about 80 people who's names I felt I should know. These were my colleagues and the anaesthetic and recovery assistants. I decided to keep it manageable by putting the surgical assistants aside for later attention. I then hung an A4 on the noticeboard in the recovery and anaesthetic team office, stating that I wanted to learn their names, and that they could help me if I made photos of them with my iPhone. This was very much appreciated. With the exception of 4 people who didn't want to be photographed, I now have the whole team in a private folder with the names as captions. This has really worked well. It still happens that I have a quick look when I am unsure, but after about two weeks I had most of the 80 names in my head. It cost some effort, but proved to be an excellent way of starting off my intensive working relationship with them. I no longer have to say, twenty times a day, "Ummm you there" or "umm what's your name again?" My surgical colleagues are not immune to this effect either; they like being called by their Christian names, and often respond the next time with mine. Using someone's first name is a small part of building the relationship, and good relationships are the basis of a friction free interaction.

Take home message:

It is well worth making the effort to learn the names of people you work with. They will value you the more for it, and it makes them more motivated to help you. I can highly recommend the "iPhone" method.

We are here on earth to do good to
others. What the others are here for, I
don't know

W.H. Auden

Talking of memory.......

We tend to think of memory in a rather black-and-white way. You remember something or you forget it. We have now learned that memory is far more complex. It would seem that when we remember something, we do not access a complete encapsulated something, consisting of sounds, pictures and feelings. Rather we assemble a memory from discrete fragments. Often we include things that we consider would have been part of the memory, but were not. An example was a study in which participants had to wait in an office before being picked up by a researcher. They were then asked questions about the office. One question was, "Was there a bookcase in the office". Most people could remember the bookcase, although there wasn't one present. The explanation is that one would expect an office to have a bookcase, so the participants found one from some other memory, and included it in their memory of the office (like cut and paste in a document).

A second example of false memory is frequently mentioned. People were asked where they were when the twin towers attack took place. Most people, including me, have no trouble remembering this. However, it turns out that many people give an answer that, when checked, was incorrect.

It would appear that we build our memories anew from the available building blocks. In this way they change with time, and are open to being manipulated. The most shocking examples of this for me are when people in a therapeutic session "remember" being abused as children. The consequences can be devastating for all concerned, and it is often not possible to prove the question one way or another. One high profile incident took place in the Netherlands (the Bolderkar affair), when some psychologists found an alarmingly high incidence of sexual abuse by parents at a kindergarten. A controversial method with a doll with sexual organs was used. Thirteen children were taken from their families and put into care. The fathers were accused, and the interviews were so harsh that three fathers even admitted to incest, whilst later found to be innocent. At the end of the day, the whole thing collapsed for lack of evidence.

In a second incident, also in the Netherlands, a mother found blood in the underpants of her four year old son. A visit to the GP suggested sexual abuse, carried out by someone in a clown suit. In no time, there were 70 other claims of sexual abuse, all by clowns! A thorough investigation led to no evidence at all.

We live in a time in which claims of sexual abuse by celebrities fill newspaper columns. Some of these cases will be genuine, some may just be getting onto a lucrative "bandwagon" and I bet a number will be people who clearly remembered something that just never happened.

Much research has been done into the question of false memories, and it is clear that it is possible in a large proportion of people to implant memories of incidents which never happened. The problem is that it is quite often impossible to pull real and false memories apart, and of course proving one's innocence can be just as hard. When these cases come into a court of law, it can be quite impossible to determine the truth. The case of the US supreme court nominee Brett Kavanaugh in 2018 is a perfect example.

In the same line, we can consider the case of witness statements after a crime. We know now that these can be wildly inaccurate, and that within five minutes after witnessing a crime, witnesses can give conflicting accounts of what they "remember". In the USA alone, there are hundreds of recorded cases of people being wrongly imprisoned for up to thirty years before their innocence was eventually proven, often by DNA analysis.

This may seem rather depressing, but there is a positive side to it all. Many people are troubled by traumatic memories, some to the point of being incapacitated. Maybe you are already ahead of me - is it possible to manipulate these memories in such a way that they lose their grip? This would appear to be the case. Before jumping on this as unethical, it's good to consider that the original memories are themselves often not accurate, and that there is something to be said for replacing disempowering inaccurate memories with empowering inaccurate ones.

It has been shown that immediately after recalling something, there is a short window of time in which the memory is malleable. This finding is used in some forms of treatment for Post traumatic stress disorder. It is called re-consolidation therapy. This therapy is in its early days, and cannot be considered to be a proven treatment yet; however, it makes sense to me.

It has also been shown that some people who do <u>not</u> develop Post traumatic stress disorder are those who have modified their memories in the years thereafter.

Take home message:

Memory remains a fascinating topic. Accept that your memory, and other people's memories are less reliable than you might expect.

Forgiving does not erase the bitter past.
A healed memory is not a deleted
memory. Instead, forgiving what we
cannot forget creates a new way to
remember.
We change the memory of our past into
a hope for our future

Lewis B. Smedes

Giving and taking criticism

Whether it was giving or taking, criticism has been a challenge for me throughout most of my career. I was rather like a eunuch in a harem; he knows exactly how it should be done, but he can't do it himself. Only in the last years have I started to become more comfortable with it.

Very often we see criticism as a personal attack and sometimes it is and sometimes it isn't. The higher our self-esteem, the less we feel the need to be reactive. When we feel attacked our natural reaction is to hit back. Generally speaking this does not work very well, but it happens before you have had time to think; as if a trigger has been pulled.

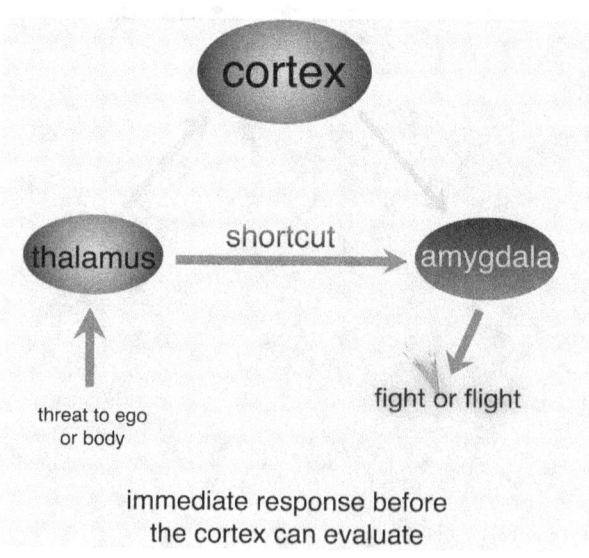

immediate response before
the cortex can evaluate

There is evidence showing that our brain's first reaction to criticism is that it is perceived as a threat just as real as a physical attack. The threat is to the ego instead of the body. The perceptions are shunted immediately to the amygdala leading to the typical fight or flight reaction.

58

(This description is useful to explain the dynamics, even if it is a gross simplification.)

"Counting to ten" is as old as the hills, but still very good advice here. And in this pause, you can consider that it is usually about something you have said or done, not about who you are — it is about behaviour, not identity. By not reacting immediately as a knee-jerk reaction, you give the higher brain centres a chance to evaluate the situation, and give a more nuanced reaction.

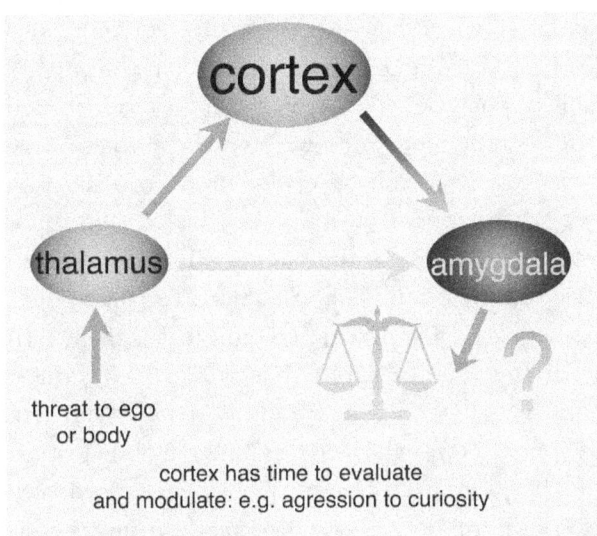

threat to ego
or body

cortex has time to evaluate
and modulate: e.g. agression to curiosity

The second thought can be, "Do I recognise anything in this criticism?" if you do, use it as feedback, and learn from it. If you don't, let it go like water off a duck's back. If it's something you can learn from, be thankful to the person who gave you this chance instead of being angry because they attacked you.

It is easier said than done and what should one do with people who do intend a personal attack? Such people are around, and they enjoy putting others down. Their motivation is probably a matter of cutting off other people's heads in order to feel a little taller. If the attack is disguised as factual criticism, then it is a good idea to question them in an open way: "tell me more about that," or "what would you hope that I shall do with that information?" Very often what they are doing is showing passive aggression. The aim is to make you look silly. As such people are usually conflict-averse the best option may be to take them aside, and say, "Have I done anything to offend you, that you make such remarks?" This has to be said in an open

59

way — you need to genuinely want to know what's behind it. It is worth taking a little time to realise that it is probably more about them than about you. What they are really communicating is that <u>they</u> have a problem; realising this makes it possible to see them more with compassion than with anger.

Often such people cause us to react emotionally: we feel hurt or angry for instance. If it is a recurring problem, some other tactics may be useful. One effective way is to make use of the fact that we make spatial representations of the people around us. Make a picture of the other person in your mind's eye. Usually you will be able to point out where they are in the space around you. They may be close, or far away, higher or lower, more to the left or the right, or right in front of you. Once you have this image, you can play around with it and notice what happens to your emotional reaction. For instance, pick that image up, and squeeze it until the person becomes very small. Then place the image further away. You will almost certainly notice that the emotional reaction weakens immediately, and this makes them easier to deal with in a balanced way. Another approach is to take what is called second and third position. Step out of your shoes, as it were, and into theirs. Then look back at yourself through their eyes, and see if that offers any insights. Then take the position of an observer, looking down on both of you from above, (third position) and see what's going on from the outside, as it were. These exercises are fun, and often lead to new insights.

It is also often useful to examine our self-image in situations in which we do not feel relaxed. We can then project an image of our "self" into the space around us, and manipulate it by making it larger and smaller, and closer or more distant. This is also fun and informative at the same time. More on this can be found in the "social panorama" model of my friend the psychologist and NLP trainer Lucas Derks.

Giving criticism

Giving criticism in a way that doesn't cause a knee jerk reaction is an art. The first thing to do is to ask yourself *why* you are going to give criticism in the first place. You need to have the expectation that what you are about to say will lead to a positive change. It is important that you aim at the level of behaviour and not identity. In other words, criticism for the sake of criticism is a waste of time and effort, and will certainly lead to a deterioration in the relationship. If someone is a complete idiot, taking the trouble to point that out is not a very useful exercise.

Having decided that something needs to be said, the next question is how. A good starting point is that people who don't comply when they are told to do something may very likely react quite differently to a request for help. If you have told your teenage son five times that he must fix the lights on his bike, a sixth attempt is unlikely to be successful. On the other hand, you could say, "I worry about you on your bicycle in the dark. I should hate anything to happen to you. You would help me feel much better if you fixed your lights." No guarantees of course, but it is more likely to be successful than the first approach.

An example from my own work is when an assistant is regularly too late in giving the instruction to bring the next patient to the holding area for a block anaesthetic. If I am angry with my assistant, I am more likely to make him or her nervous and uncertain. It will probably lead to a deterioration in the quality of the help I get rather than an improvement. On the other hand, if I ask for help, then I am very likely to get it. I could point out that it is very important to me to set my blocks early because they then work better; and if I do it at the last minute, the surgical team has to wait for me, and I find that stressful. I also hate it when my block has too little time to work properly and I have to give the patient a general anaesthetic after all. This is far more likely to change the behaviour of my assistant, and instead of damaging the relationship it actually strengthens it by underlining that he is important to me. So the best solution is to present the situation as your problem, and point out that they can help you with it.

61

Take home message

Improving our skills in giving and taking criticism will directly lead to a more satisfying life and improve our effectiveness in all areas in which we have to deal with other people. Whether criticism is meant kindly or maliciously, the approach is the same: take time before reacting, and then use curiosity to find if there is a kernel of truth from which we can learn and grow.

> It ain't what you don't know that gets you into trouble. It's what you know for sure that just ain't so

Mark Twain

Jumping to conclusions

In an Irish pub, one of the older customers had a strange habit; he would come to the bar and order three pints of beer. He would then take them to the back of the room where he sat alone at a small table with the three beers distributed over its surface. He would then drink them one at a time. This happened at the start of every month. Eventually the bar-keeper plucked up the courage to ask him what it was about. "Oh," he said, "I have two brothers, one lives in Toronto and one in Cape Town. To give us the feeling that we are still in contact we agreed that on the same day each month we would go to a pub and in this way have a drink with each other. Sounds a bit sentimental I know, but we like doing it". Satisfied, the bar keeper returned to his bar, and watched the ritual repeat itself each month for a couple of years. Then on one occasion the man came in and ordered just two pints, and went to his usual place. The bar-keeper was a little sentimental himself, and he felt for the man. So he went over and said, "I couldn't help seeing that you only ordered two pints; I'm so sorry." The man looked up puzzled and then burst out laughing. "No, no, there's nothing wrong — my brothers are fine. It's just that I've given up alcohol myself"

So this chapter is about jumping to conclusions. This is something most of us are expert in; and we need to be. I'll come to that in a moment, but first here is another little example.

Look for a moment at the figure below, and then with your eyes closed, repeat to yourself what you have seen.

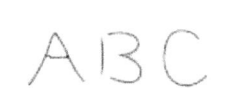

Most people have no problem doing this. You will also probably know that the letters were on the left, and the numbers on the right. You may also have formed an image of Ann approaching the bank in your mind's eye. What very few people see is the ambiguity in the illustration. Are there three letters on the left, or two letters and a number? If you look carefully you will see that the 13 and the B are identical. People will swear to what they have seen, and be prepared to start a war for what they 'know' is right, to stretch the point a little. This is what the quote above from Mark Twain is referring to. In the same way, the image of Ann you conjured up may be of her approaching a financial bank, or the bank of a river. Very few will stop long enough to think of possible alternatives.

Our unconscious mind is lightening quick, and offers an immediate interpretation of what we have in front of us. Our conscious mind generally just goes happily along with this interpretation. This is at the same time essential to our survival and a great pitfall. If we tried to evaluate all possible interpretations of what we experience, we should likely go mad, while our split second decisions are usually spot on. Because our decisions are generally trustworthy we also become lazy. The result is that, if you stood to win a million on the lottery ticket with the winning combination A13C (as written above), you would not bother to claim it (which may or may not be a bad thing)!

There is a very important lesson in this for us; when it comes down to decisions that are going to have a big influence on us, then it is vital that after we have drawn our conclusions, we take a time out, and ask ourselves if we could have drawn another conclusion from the same situation. Another small anecdote may illustrate this.

A small boy comes downstairs after happily playing in the bath with his toy submarine. Shortly after his mother accuses him angrily of peeing beside the toilet pot. The child proclaims his innocence, but his mother points to the damning evidence of the puddle surrounding the pot. Father decides to take a look, and sees that the steam in the bathroom has caused condensation on the old-fashioned water reservoir above the toilet. This has dripped onto the floor, creating the puddle. You may well think that this is a minor matter, but if you take a moment to step into the little boy's slippers, you will see that he had unjustly been accused of lying. At such a tender age, this only has to be repeated a few times to cause real damage to the trusting relationship between parent and child.

If you are like me, you will be able to come up with examples when you caused damage to a relationship by jumping to the wrong conclusion.

The message is; this is going to happen to you again and you can mitigate the damage by being aware of this phenomenon, and asking yourself, "Is there another possible explanation that would put this in another (more positive) light?

Next time you are driving in a hurry, and the little man with a hat on in the tiny car in front of you is pushing your blood pressure up by driving at a snail's pace, ask yourself, "Could it be that he hasn't driven the car for five years, and his wife is now sick in the hospital and he is on the way to visit her?" Maybe it isn't true, but just considering the possibility will almost certainly have a moderating effect on your blood pressure.

Take home message

Just being aware that jumping to conclusions is a normal part of being human, helps us to be more mild in our judgement of ourselves and others when it happens. Stopping to ask yourself if there might be another possible explanation is a valuable exercise and may lead you to ask questions instead of letting your conclusion become set in concrete.

Even very young children need to be informed about dying. Explain the concept of death very carefully to your child. This will make threatening him with it much more effective

P.J. O'Rourke

We all want to be heard

To illustrate what I mean, let me give an anecdote; it occurred on the day before I started writing this chapter. In my hospital I regularly have to work with a plastic surgeon who is also of retirement age, and also shows no sign of wanting to stop. As far as I can see he does his work well, but he is, shall we say, not the most fun colleague to work with. He rarely smiles, generally looks grumpy, says little and reacts to questions as if he would rather not be bothered.

Yesterday one of my patients was a twelve year old girl for a hand operation. I chatted to her and her mother and we came to the conclusion that a nerve block of her arm, with a bit of sedation would be a good option. We carried out the block with the girl lightly sedated and mother next to her. When we set off to the operating theatre, my assistant warned me that the surgeon was angry because he considered the child too young to have a nerve block.

How should one react at such a moment in order to change the surgeon's mind, and improve the working relationship?

I approached him and the following discussion ensued, "I understand you find this girl too young for a block?" "Yes." "Can you tell me what your reasoning is for thinking that?" (better than "why," which often elicits a defensive reaction). "It's very traumatic for a child." "Ok, I quite agree with you that we must use the least traumatic techniques with children. I think that if you speak to the mother later you will find that the procedure was in no way traumatic for her. It's not so much what we do as how we do it that counts." "And I often hear that patients hate the feeling of a sleeping arm all day." "Yes, I hear that sometimes as well. On the other hand, I want this girl to arrive on the recovery ward with no pain, and no need of morphine injections which are also not pleasant and can make her vomit and feel dizzy." "Ok, that's true as well". End of discussion. You may bet that I instructed my assistant that if the girl gave the slightest whimper during the operation, she was to knock her out with a hammer, needs be. This was going to be an exemplary anaesthetic in the surgeon's eyes and I am happy to report that the hammer was not necessary.

Later on the surgeon was carrying out a procedure for a breast reconstruction after cancer; a technique that was new to me. I asked him about it, and he started talking, ending with a site on the internet where I could find more information. I visited the site, and it was very interesting. Later I talked further with him about it, and it was as if I had a different person in front of me. I expect that next time we work together, we shall both enjoy the experience more.

So what happened here? I could have reacted in a number of ways. One option was to ignore his comments; after all, the choice of anaesthetic was not his business. However, approaching him and addressing the subject directly compels a degree of respect. I could have reacted with irritation and said that he should not comment like that to my assistant. I could have said he was wrong and that it was not traumatic for the child. What I did was to choose curiosity as my tool; curiosity has the double advantage of giving the other person the feeling that you are interested in their opinion. This is very disarming. On top of that it gives you new information which may or may not be valuable, and at any rate something you can react to instead of just entering into an "Is!" "Isn't!" sort of discussion.

What I also did was to tell him he was right where I could. We tend to view people who tell us we are right are very insightful people; probably intelligent and more likeable. (This is one of our unconscious triggers; it is so ingrained that there is almost no getting round it.) So I agreed with him where I could — we should avoid traumatising our patients, and some people do complain about the dead feeling in the arm. Now that I am insightful and more likeable, it may even be the case that I am worth listening to!

After that I expressed (a genuine) interest in his work. This combination of listening, agreeing and showing interest is an almost irresistible approach (like honey for Winnie the Pooh).

I can imagine that some readers will react by saying that I am just being manipulative, or a sycophant and that they are not going to waste their time on someone who shows no empathy at all and is generally seen as a pain in the neck.

We cannot interact with other people <u>without</u> influencing them in some way; if I had reacted angrily in this situation I should have "manipulated" the surgeon into giving a negative reaction. What you can do is to <u>choose</u> the way you influence people to get the result you want; if this results in a better and happier working relationship for both in the future, then I am all for manipulation!

In this case the result of the interaction could only be improved mutual respect, a more pleasurable working relationship and better patient care. Everyone wins. And who knows, once people start coming out of their shells they may even become fun to work with. Key to all this is that your curiosity and your interest both need to be genuine; if they are not, it is just a trick, and people are quick to see through it.

Take home message

The title of an earlier chapter covers this sufficiently: try first to understand, and then to be understood.

Our doubts are traitors, and make us lose the good we oft might win by fearing to attempt.

William Shakespeare

Assertiveness and bullies

V ery few of us get any formal training in assertiveness. For many people it has a negative connotation. However, someone who is going to work and train in the world of doctors is going to need it.

A classic example of this was an interaction with a woman surgeon I worked with. She was one of the very first female surgeons in the Netherlands. She was a good and dedicated doctor, but in some way very vulnerable. She came across as hard as nails, and if she had an assistant who she didn't trust, she could make life for that assistant most unpleasant. On one occasion she had caused a young theatre nurse to burst into tears during an operation. When I tackled her about it after the operation, she burst into tears herself! She was as soft as butter inside. Nonetheless, I find it unforgivable how surgeons will often vent their frustrations on the least assertive of their assistants. I gave the nurse in question a mini assertiveness training, which she applied to good effect not only with that surgeon, but also in her further career. With training I just mean a ten minute talk about body language, telling the doctor how her behaviour made her feel, approaching the doctor without delay, and with no one other present and showing how vulnerable she felt. I worked with her for years and was gratified to see how she stood up to the doctors, and was treated with respect as a result. Such a small intervention, and such a great and long-lasting result. Of course, here I am patting myself on the back, but it is important to be humble enough to realise that she might have become assertive of her own accord, with my intervention being irrelevant.

Aside: This, by the way, is true of many medical interventions. A patient has a sore throat, we give an antibiotic and the patient gets better. We think we are very clever, but of course the patient most likely would have got better without the antibiotic, and without the negative effects antibiotics can have. Patients often get better; sometimes as a result of the treatment, and sometimes despite it.

Another example of the benefits of assertiveness was an orthopaedic surgeon I worked with who carried out operations in two hospitals. In one he was a horror; throwing instruments, including knives, was not exceptional. In the other hospital he was as meek as a lamb. I asked the theatre head in the hospital where he behaved himself for an explanation. "Simple," she said, "We don't tolerate that sort of behaviour from anyone."

In private life this surgeon was a normal, friendly person. In a situation in which he felt personally threatened or uncertain — a difficult operation, for instance — he reverted to a primitive version of himself.

In general bullies are weak, and cover their weakness with aggression. If you say, "boo" loud enough, they will usually run away.

Many nurses and junior staff are afraid that an assertive approach might endanger their position. This fear is usually (but not always) unfounded. The clue is to react to bullying in the right place, with the right words and at the right time.

The right place is where you can be alone with the bully. Attempting to correct him in the presence of others will damage an already threatened ego, and almost certainly lead to an unpleasant scene. The right time is as soon as the dust has settled, and both of you have calmed down. If it is not done at once, then the chance is great that it will not be done at all (postponing ≡ cancelling). The right words are not words of criticism, but words explaining what his behaviour does to you, and an appeal for help.

For instance you could start by saying, "Dr. A, when you talk to me the way you did during the operation, you make me feel (uncertain, angry, disrespected, sad etc). It makes it harder for me to assist you in the way I should like to. I should be much obliged if you would take this into account in the future." This is assertiveness; you avoid direct criticism, you stay calm and polite, you make clear the effect of his behaviour on you, and you ask him to take account of this in the future. Do not expect a miracle; it may be hard for the other to react in a healthy way at that moment. However it is almost certain that he will modify his behaviour in the future.

If this all seems too circuitous to you, and you want a quick fix and don't feel too vulnerable, then if a surgeon explodes during an operation you could say, "When you are prepared to communicate normally, we can continue this discussion." Or "would you mind finding another outlet for your frustrations?" However, it should be remembered that the doctor is probably already under stress, and it may not be in the interest of the patient to make matters worse. Better would be, "I will (not) do what you ask, and I should like to talk with you alone after the operation." By the time you talk, things will already be shifting in his head. He knows what's coming, and he knows you are right, and you will have calmed down (maybe to the point that you regret saying anything! But don't back down; this little confrontation will spare you much frustration in the future, and will certainly lead to the surgeon treating you with more respect henceforth). It goes without saying that he and him can just as easily be replaced with she and her.

Just the other day I worked with an ENT surgeon and an inexperienced anaesthetic assistant. Toward the end of the programme the ENT surgeon commented that all five of the patients up until then had shown some movement during the operation. None of the patients would have noticed this, but movement is a nuisance for any surgeon, and especially for an ENT surgeon, when, during a delicate ear operation for example, it can be disastrous. No surgeon wants to follow their patient into the next room in order to complete the operation! It was interesting to watch the interaction. The surgeon did not make his remarks in an aggressive way, but the assistant shot into defence mode, explaining that he had given the correct dosage and was just following instructions, etc. This was not an assertive reaction; he gave no recognition at all to the fact that the surgeon had experienced problems that were our responsibility to prevent. He could simply have said, "I'm sorry that you have been having problems; patients shouldn't move. I guess we haven't scored very well today and I shall see whether there is anything I should have done differently, and try to avoid it in the future." With the first reaction the surgeon doesn't feel that he is taken seriously, and has no reason to expect that it will go better the next time. Next time he works with this assistant he will expect things to go wrong again, and we know that people tend to live up (and down!) to expectations. Unwittingly the assistant had started a downward spiral in relations and in performance. The surgeon would start thinking, "Oh, not him again!" and the assistant would be aware of this and his own negative thoughts which would set him up to fail.

I am going into some detail here, and it may seem as if I am blowing a tiny incident out of proportion. What I want to make clear is that our relationships and performance are the sum of all these little incidents, and that we have a choice; use an assertive approach, dare to be vulnerable, and make sure that your slope goes uphill. The assistant should have seen this incident and the surgeon's remarks as feedback, not as failure. Seeing it as failure made him unhappy, uncertain, defensive and almost certainly put him on the path to the next "failure".

In this case I took over the assertive/vulnerable bit, and we had a constructive conversation with the surgeon, increasing our mutual understanding. Hopefully I was teaching by example, but I should really have spent some time after the programme, to explain all this to the assistant. Because most people know <u>when</u> things are going wrong, but are unaware <u>why</u>, and how to put it right.

Take-home message

Let's change — "You did something wrong, therefore you are stupid or incompetent" into — " It didn't go as it should, did it? Can we have a look at what went wrong and how we could prevent this another time?" The first approach only leads to defensiveness and deteriorating quality of work. With the second you will see that people are prepared to talk of their mistakes, which is part of learning not to repeat them. This openness and non-blaming is essential in our profession, and very often we ourselves are the cause of blocking it.

Be the kind of woman that when your feet hit the floor each morning the devil says,
"Oh crap, she's up"

Anon

Keep your hands off me

Sexual intimidation is of all times and places. The predator is almost always a man, and the worst cases are associated with men in a position of power, and women in a vulnerable position. Hospitals in particular present many opportunities for harassment. For instance, a medical specialist who has the power to make or break the career of a trainee doctor. Or simply because the difference in status makes it hard for someone to behave assertively. In a recent study in Belgium, about one in three residents reported that they had been approached inappropriately on at least one occasion. One reported being in a room with staff members and other juniors on her first day, and one of the staff members asked them all to write their cup size on the blackboard. The question is tasteless enough, but what is really disturbing is that there was no one present who raised their voice to say that it was inappropriate (see the chapter on herd instinct and culture). It is quite possible that most present saw it as a bit of innocent fun. This makes it a difficult subject to deal with.

There is something about hospitals and doctors that seems to play into this theme. There are, for instance, innumerable doctor's romances, and television series about doctors and hospitals in which romance plays an inevitable role and the doctor with his status is the object of adoration. We are back to the doctor's ego again. Maybe this long history creates an atmosphere in which it is considered normal for doctors to have a physical relationship with subordinates.

Defining sexual harassment is not a clear cut matter, but simply stated, sexual intimidation is present if someone *feels* sexually intimidated. It is not sufficient for the perpetrator to say, "I thought she enjoyed it" or, "it was just an innocent bit of fun". If someone feels that they have been violated, then that is the criterium. This does not always imply that the perpetrator had any sexual intentions, or meant any harm. But their behaviour has caused another to *feel* that they have been harassed, and that behaviour needs to stop.

The definition is complicated by the fact that some women may actively enjoy exactly the same behaviour, or even provoke it. Some women will certainly use their physical attractiveness as a means to promotion. Where one may feel flattered at the attention, and another may see it as just an innocent bit of flirting, for some it is highly unpleasant and intimidating. So we can speak of wanted and unwanted intimacy and our concern here is with the second sort.

Because there may be innocent misunderstandings, it is essential that the "victim" makes clear that the attention is unwanted, and a pre-requisite for doing so is that the culture makes it possible without fear of reprisals.

Sexual harassment may take different forms: unwanted touching, sexually explicit language, pornographic images, gestures, etc. The most extreme form is probably, "You want to keep your job/get promotion? Sleep with me."

I worked in a hospital where there was a colleague who regularly pushed the limits of what is appropriate, without it being egregious. He tried it with an anaesthetic assistant once. She made it quite clear that it was unwelcome, and it never happened again with her. However, others were too afraid to stand up to him, and were the subject of repeated unwelcome touching. The assistants observed that the same doctor usually did not take the trouble to listen to the heart and lungs of patients, but that he was particularly conscientious when it came to girls and young women. When one patient complained about feeling violated by his examination, he was reported to the head of department — he had crossed a threshold. I never heard of this particular behaviour being repeated.

The question arises of who's responsibility it is to prevent such behaviour. I think that it is a shared responsibility.

The perpetrator: men in a position of power should be well aware that sexual advances or language may be unwelcome, and also how hard it can be for a person in a vulnerable situation to address this. They have a responsibility to avoid harming others. However, there are many people with psychopathic tendencies, and this argument will be meaningless to them.

The victim. Victims of sexual harassment often say nothing because they are afraid of the consequences. My experience is that it is vitally important that they inform the perpetrator that his advances are unwelcome. To start with, it is unfair not to — it may be that the man really wasn't aware of the effect of what he was doing, or that her colleagues enjoy his attention, and he assumed she would. "Dr. I'm sure you don't mean any harm, but when you touch me like that I feel really uncomfortable." A very important point here is clarity. When I am sailing, and I see the possibility of a collision with another vessel, I can change course just enough to avoid that. But far better is to make an unnecessarily large change of course, so that the other sailor has no doubt about my intentions. Otherwise, they may also make a small change of course which could lead to the collision we were trying to avoid. "Don't do that please" is far more effective that an embarrassed shrug. A decent man will apologise, and the issue is solved. I am sure that this is more effective than reporting the incident to a departmental head. To start with, it creates respect, which doesn't happen when a woman goes behind his back to the chief, and it fundamentally changes the relationship into a more equal one. It also avoids unnecessarily harming the perpetrator, and gives him a chance to change his behaviour. If however the behaviour is repeated, then the next step is to protest more forcefully: "If you do that again, would you prefer a slap in the face, or that I report the incident to the head of department?" Unfortunately such a hard approach is unthinkable for many, and I think that that is a pity; when dealing with bullies, nothing works better than standing up to them in no uncertain terms. Unfortunately, just as with bullies in general, it is the weaker ones who get picked on, and they are the ones who dare not create a fuss. Many victims are scared that it will cost them their job; it is possible, but I think that that is very rare in a hospital situation, and losing your integrity out of fear is seldom a good idea. If the behaviour doesn't stop after that, then it is time to report the matter.

The head of department. The head of department has a responsibility for the behaviour of his staff, the culture within his department and the security of personnel in lower echelons.

In an individual case, the head first needs to be aware. Obviously, if it is not brought to his attention, he will not be able to act. Part of his responsibility is to ensure that he has the trust of workers at all levels, and that he is approachable. It is very easy for the head of department, often bound up in meetings, and less present on the shop floor, to lose touch; especially with those lower in the hierarchy. If the head is seen as distant and unapproachable, then such signals will come late. I well remember the director of one of the hospitals I worked in, who would regularly turn up on a department just for a chat with the staff. He picked signals up early as a result, which gave him the chance to intervene before a situation got out of hand. (He didn't often come to the operating theatres, though - I think that scared him!)

The head has two ways to approach such a situation — general and specific. In general the staff should know that there is a zero-tolerance policy toward sexual harassment in the department; this point of view could be a topic during a staff meeting, and new staff members could be informed of this fact when they are taken on.

The head may also create opportunities for subordinate staff to learn how they can best cope with such situations, through a training session, possibly with specially trained actors to practise with. In the Netherlands there are calls for every person entering medical training to receive instruction on this topic.

Specifically the head can speak to the accused, and hear his side of the story. This is important; the other side of a story can be surprising! The message could then be, "I'm saying nothing about your intentions, but I am saying that at least one worker experienced it as sexual intimidation.

80

Whether that lies in your insensitivity or her hyper-sensitivity is neither here nor there - I am just asking you to modify your behaviour, and to be aware that some people feel that you go to far."

A zero-tolerance policy implies sanctions; if these are not there, the perpetrator does not have to take the warning very seriously. The head needs to be explicit about what the consequences will be. That said, in many cases the shame associated with being reported, spoken to by the head of department and having a remark added to your dossier is sufficient to prevent recurrence.

A mediation meeting between accused and victim may be clarifying and healing. In the Netherlands most larger hospitals have a confidential counsellor. This is an official who is independent, and can be consulted in confidence. They may be approached by anyone. A head of department could ask such a person to act as mediator, or an official mediator may be employed. The head could act as mediator himself, as long as both parties are completely happy with this.

Blackmail. I understand that it is very easy for me to give this advice. Someone who is a single parent, and completely dependent on her job for her living and that of her children, may make the calculation that the risks are too high. They may choose to do nothing. Sometimes they may make this choice not because the risk is so great, but because it is an excuse not to be assertive.

False accusations. Of course blackmail works in two directions. When a specialist threatens a junior with blocking their career if they object to his advances, then one response might be considered appropriate under the circumstances: "Yes doctor, I am vulnerable and dependent on you for my future. But you are also vulnerable. If a frustrated junior, who has just missed a deserved promotion, were to make a false claim that you had raped her in the hospital lift, then that would probably be the end of your career."

Why do I even mention such a course of action? I think that it is my frustration at the thought that this problem is so often seen as an unavoidable fact of life. False accusations are rare, but they do happen. The head of department should be aware of this, and listen to the complaint empathically, and critically. If a member of staff who has a strong record of ethical behaviour toward juniors gets one complaint, then extra vigilance is called for.

Take home message

After more than 40 years experience, I have seen much. My conclusion is that the very best way to deal with sexual harassment is for the victim to approach the perpetrator, preferably alone (unless physical violence is a real possibility) and to be *very* clear about what his behaviour is doing to her. And this is important — no blaming, but clearly telling him how it affects her. In a way, she is asking for his help, instead of attacking him. This approach is far more effective, and less likely to elicit anger and aggression. By doing this, the victim compels the perpetrator to respect her, and it changes their relationship in a positive way. This does not happen when she complains to a higher-up without giving the perpetrator the chance to correct it himself. This step should be reserved for when a direct appeal does not work.

> Either this man is dead, or my watch
> has stopped.

Groucho Marx

Ambition, criteria and goals

This chapter is to explain why it is important to have goals, to choose your goals wisely and to avoid the pitfalls of choosing goals for the wrong reasons.

Ambition and goals are overlapping terms. Ambition may be seen as a more general form of a goal. For instance, an ambition may be: "I want to become a powerful and influential person." A goal could be, "I shall start by becoming Head of the student union."

Goals are very important to achieving a full and satisfying life, and there is an easy explanation for this. Our minds are bombarded with a mass of information the whole day long. We simply do not have the mental processing power to pay attention to it all. If we try, we go mad. This is one problem for people with schizophrenia — they have trouble sifting irrelevant information out. Therefore our minds need a system to help us focus our attention on relevant things. Part of this process is the reticular activating system (RAS). I can explain its function by the following example.

Your favourite uncle has died and left you his old Citroen 2CV, the apple of his eye. Up until now you have considered these cars as amongst the ugliest and least interesting you have ever seen. Now it suddenly takes on a new emotional significance, and without your having to do anything, you start seeing 2CV's wherever you go. It is as if a gate has been opened, and these cars have escaped and are now everywhere. Your RAS is waving a little flag every time and saying, "Here is another of those cars you have become interested in". In the past it would just have ignored them.

I am writing here about selective attention, and if you haven't already seen it, I can highly recommend that you check out "the monkey business illusion" video by Daniel Simons on YouTube; it has become a classic.

84

If we have no goals, our RAS just has no idea what it should be looking out for (yes, it knows that driving through red lights is a bad idea, so it flags them as well). The moment you set a goal, and make it important to you, your RAS will start working for you, and will pick things out of the background chaos which might be relevant to achieving this goal. If you are interested in learning chess, your RAS will point out to you a piece in the paper about the setting up of a local chess club which you would simply not have seen otherwise.

In short, our minds need us to give them direction, and then they will happily work away for us in the background. No direction means that the thoughts in our minds will blow about in any direction the wind takes them. That is why we need to set goals.

Good goals and bad goals

Ambition is often defined in one of two ways: a desire to achieve a particular aim, or: an eager or strong desire to achieve power, fame, wealth or rank. This second case is in my opinion where it all goes wrong. Whereas setting and achieving a goal, such as, "I want to be a really good surgeon" can lead to a life of great satisfaction, goals like power, fame, wealth or rank rarely do so. Many politicians are moved by such motives, but it is known that "great" politicians rarely die great. Take the example of the British prime minister Tony Blair. After riding the wave of success he now has enormous wealth, but is despised by many of the people who put him for a short time on his throne.

It is not that there is anything inherently wrong with things like power, fame and wealth. I wouldn't mind a bit more of those myself. It goes wrong when those things are your primary goal because they simply will not make you happy. There is ample evidence that this is true. If your primary goal is to make things better for society, and you think that you can achieve this through politics, you may just get all the trappings of high office and become happy doing it.

I am afraid however that many people who started out with high ideals end up disillusioned as they get sucked into a life in which straightforward honesty loses out to power play and political conniving. Maybe I'm over cynical, but I fear that if you were to put all the top leaders the world has known together, you would not find many acting out of altruistic motives, and I suspect not many will be well balanced and happy individuals. Let us not forget the famous words of Lord Acton, "Power tends to corrupt, and absolute power corrupts absolutely. Great men are almost always bad men."

So if your ambition is for a position of power or influence, such as becoming a professor of a medical department, make sure first that your ambition is fed by motives which may make you happy. Unfortunately, many people in such positions are motivated by the need to shore up feelings of inadequacy. Their motivation has a direct influence on the lives and happiness of the people who serve under them.

I hope that I have made it clear in the beginning of this chapter that having goals and going after them is essential to growth and happiness. Unfortunately many people either have no clearly defined goals, or they choose goals which will not bring them happiness and fulfilment. We need a way to choose our goals wisely, and here are a number of criteria:

Prerequisites for a good goal:

- Is it stated in the positive?

- Is it a goal of your own choosing?

- Is it achievable through your own effort?

- Is there a clear context (where, when, how and with whom, will I be doing my goal)?

- Is it realistic? — The goal of becoming the first man on the moon is no longer realistic (unless you believe in conspiracy theories!)

- Do I have the resources necessary? Which extra resources do I need to pick up to achieve the goal?

- Is it measurable? (it is important to know when you have arrived, as it were. What will I be doing when I have achieved it? What will I be seeing, thinking, feeling)

- Is it timed? (you need to set a time frame for achieving it)

- Is it ecological? (achieving the goal must not harm the interests of yourself or others). These questions are important: Why do I really want this goal? What will I lose and what will I gain if I achieve it? What will happen if I achieve it? What will happen if I don't achieve it?

- Is it clear what the first step will be, and when? (Lao Tzu: a journey of a thousand miles begins with a single step)

When stating goals, the importance of stating it in the positive cannot be over stressed. It is said that the unconscious mind does not process negatives. Thus, "don't drop that" may be seen as an invitation to drop it. I once saw the British celebrity Derren Brown talking to a top tightrope walker in negatives; don't look down! Don't think about falling! And indeed he eventually fell, for the first time in his career, I believe.

"I want to stop smoking" is less empowering than, "I want to become a non-smoker". "My wife wants me to stop smoking" is a real non-starter — negative and not of your own choosing.

A well formed goal

Here is an example of choosing a goal. It is to become an amateur tennis player who can play well at club level.

- It is stated in the positive

- It is something I want

- It is achievable through my own effort

87

- The context is clear - I shall be playing in my local club with friends and other members

- It is realistic — they are taking on new members, and I have free time

- Resources - I am physically fit, I can pay the membership fees. I need added resources and shall have to take tennis lessons, buy a racket, etc.

- It is measurable - I can take part in tournaments and measure my progress

- It can be timed - I want to play my first tournament this year

- It is ecological - I shall increase my social contacts, improve my fitness, enjoy myself and hurt no one in the process.

- The first step is clear - I shall fill in the application form today

Your personal criteria

When deciding on goals, it is a good idea to stop and decide what your criteria and priorities are, and put these up against what achieving your goals will bring you. It is unfortunate that so few people stop to consider what is really important to them. They get so caught up in living their life that they don't really consider where they are heading. They just arrive somewhere and then life just seems to take over. You are so busy living it that you tend not to stop and ask yourself if this path is bringing you what you really want.

I once asked a colleague what the most important things in life were. He came back with personal happiness, physical and mental health, family and financial security. This man was working about eighty hours a week, smoking and drinking too much, taking no exercise and was chairman of the Medical board and member of a number of committees. No surprise then when he got divorced and had his first heart attack.

I don't think this man ever stopped to think whether his life-style was supporting his criteria. He had achieved financial independence, but none of the other things he knew were important. He probably never asked himself questions like, "If I could choose between a little less money, and more time with my family, what would I choose?" "If I could choose between dropping a couple of committees and spending time on my physical condition, what would I do?"

It is not possible to check whether we are living according to our criteria if we have never considered what they are, and few people do this. A little exercise would be useful to illustrate this. Take a piece of paper and write down your criteria, most important at the top. You might have health, happiness, family, financial independence, a good job etc underneath each other. Now you can take the top two, and ask yourself, "If I had to give up a little of a to get a bit more of b would I do that?" You can then do this for the whole list, and in this way refine the order. Then you may ask yourself if your life and your plans are aligned with this list. The above mentioned colleague might be alive today if he had done that.

Take-home message

If and when you become a doctor, I hope you will consider well what your goals will be, and monitor them from time to time to see that they are aligned with your criteria. Both your criteria and goals can be modified by time and experience; the important thing is that they are aligned with one another.

It's hard to fight an enemy who has
outposts in your head

Sally Kempton

90

Saying 'no'

Much of good goal setting depends on your ability not only to decide what is healthy for you but also your ability to cope with external pressure and expectations. It means being able to say "no" when you feel that something is not good for you. It means monitoring how much stress you need and can cope with. That is very personal — some people seem to thrive on working weeks which make me dizzy just to contemplate. Others have a very low stress tolerance. I am not sure that there is a lot you can do to change your optimal stress level, but it is certain that too little and too much are not good for you. If you do a job you really like, then a heavy workload will not feel so stressful. So again; do a job you love or find another!

It is of great importance that you monitor and recognise whether you are in balance in this respect, and it would be wonderful if managers and organisations were able to take account of the fact that it is not good to put the same workload on everyone. A manager can quickly run into problems if he has a group of workers in the same function, because it is almost impossible to give one vulnerable person lighter duties; the others would probably not take kindly to it, so that the lighter duties would ultimately be just as stressful because others look on you as inferior.

Problems start to accumulate when you are asked to do something that you feel in your bones is not good for you, but you cannot say "no". This may be because you are afraid of the consequences (for example losing your job) and it may be because the task will give you recognition or influence or money. Going over your limits for a short period will probably do little harm, but doing so for long periods will be damaging to your health and may lead to burn out. Many relationships fall apart through one of the partners not recognising, or not correcting this.

One way round the problem of not being able to say "no" is to say "yes" instead. Sounds pretty illogical, but maybe an example will make it clear. You work hard at a full-time job, and at the end of the week you notice that you are tired and irritable and hardly able to enjoy the weekend. You just use it to recover. Finding time and energy for your partner or children is almost too much for you. In other words, you are just about coping; the water is already up to your chin. Your boss then comes along with a project that is going to cost time and effort. You may feel unable to refuse, or maybe it is a very interesting project, but you know that taking it on would be unwise and exact a price in terms of relationships and health.

In this situation you could say, "Yes, of course I will do it." And then: "How are we going to delegate some of my other tasks while I am working on the new project?" You have said "yes" and immediately coupled your yes to a reduction in some other area. This is more effective than saying "no, I can't cope with it," and shows that you are prepared to take on new work, and also to set limits. If your boss nonetheless just says, "Do it, and no delegation" then you should think very seriously about looking for a new job. If you do not, then you are accepting conditions which are not good for you, and may lead to a burn out.

By the way, saying "yes" and then adding conditions is in general far more effective than just saying "no". It shows willingness, and that is always important to the other person. It may well turn into a "no" if the conditions are not met, but it will be far better respected.

Take-home message

Give your ambitions a regular health check, make goals that will bring you happiness and growth, make sure that criteria and activities are aligned with each other and monitor and respect your limits. Then you will have done what you can to create and maintain a life worth living.

Twenty years from now you will be more disappointed by the things that you didn't do than by the ones you did do. So throw off the bowlines. Sail away from safe harbour. Catch the trade winds in your sails.
Explore. Dream. Discover.

Mark Twain

Medical Research

the two edged sword

"Believe none of what you hear and half of what you see." I remember the name of the teacher who said this, which school, which room and where I was sitting at the time; that much of an impression it made on me. I like to think that that moment helped me to take a critical approach to life.

How much of what we believe and do in the medical world is based on facts and the truth? I fear that it is far less than we would like to believe. Some examples will make this clear.

When I trained as an anaesthetist in the late 1970's, it was standard to give all patients an injection of the drug atropine and a sedative in the "premedication" about an hour before the operation. Why the atropine? The standard answer that all anaesthetists would give me was "to dry the secretions in the airways". Why would one want to do that? The end result was always an unpleasant dry mouth for the patient, and indeed a drying of the secretions, making for thick viscous sputum, which was hard for the airway's mechanisms to remove. This could be a precipitating factor in lung infections postoperatively. So you could reasonably expect that this drying of the secretions must also have clear benefits — why else would you subject a patient to it?

Well, no, actually it did not. It <u>used</u> to in the past when we were using ether as an anaesthetic. This was so irritant to the airways that it caused a flood of secretions. Fortunately, by the time I took up anaesthetics, ether was no longer being used. My consultant at the time felt that I should be able to administer an ether anaesthetic, and so some poor man was chosen to be my victim. I am sure that he was not asked ahead of time whether this would be OK, and I am sure that if he had known how it was to have an ether anaesthetic, he would not have given permission. The ether was administered by dripping it onto a mask covered with gauze. It evaporated, and was inhaled, causing a fit of coughing and gagging. Eventually the patient slept, and the rest was uneventful. Looking back, I find the incident difficult to justify ethically; it was also the only patient in my entire career who actually benefitted from atropine in the premedication.

Since the ether period, the anaesthetic drugs no longer caused the same irritation and stimulation of sputum production. Despite this, for about 20 years thereafter patients over the whole world were still being given this drug, which was giving them no benefit, and some discomfort, or actual harm. When I questioned it, consultants would admit that the drying of secretions was no longer necessary, but that it also protected against bradycardia — an abnormal slowing of the heart rate. This was pure rationalisation — bradycardia could be far more effectively treated by injecting atropine intravenously when needed. Having received these answers, I just stopped using the drug in the pre-medication and no one noticed any difference. It's just that it spared the patients the dry mouth. It also saved money and work for the nurses.

(Ether is a safe anaesthetic requiring little in the way of equipment. It is still used in primitive settings.)

As far as I know, no clinical studies ever demonstrated the advantage of using atropine in this way, and as I write this, I realise how hard it is to believe how highly educated professionals could be so little self-critical. It was really just "we have always done it this way" and it is a great example of the importance of doing studies into the ways we work. It is just one of very many treatment methods which had been developed, but never critically compared to alternative treatments.

It is also an example of doctors who "just know" what is right and wrong. When I emigrated to the Netherlands in 1977, I started work in a teaching hospital where the second in command of the department knew a lot of things that were just "right". I shall never forget when I suggested during a staff meeting that it might be an idea to start pre-medicating patients orally — tablets in place of injections. This man subjected me to ridicule for such a stupid suggestion. The next thing I would be suggesting was that patients be allowed to eat breakfast! Well, shortly thereafter, oral premedication became the universal standard, and yes, if operated on later in the day, patients are now indeed often allowed a light breakfast. So much for "just knowing". This attitude from a person with so much influence within the department was one of the main reasons I left the university and moved to a peripheral hospital where I would have more latitude to follow and push new thinking.

Medical studies have been highly effective in innumerable cases, so that the quality of medical care today is based more and more on demonstrable facts. This is really very necessary; although most anaesthetists would claim to be "scientific" very many clinical decisions are based on emotion. One example I heard just the other day is anaesthesia for caesarian section. I had been carrying out the procedure under regional anaesthesia — a spinal or epidural anaesthetic — since 1977. By that time there was sufficient evidence, and I always felt that giving a general anaesthetic for this procedure was equivalent to theft — one took one of the most deeply significant events in the life of a woman, and by putting her to sleep, stole this moment, as it were, without any good rationale. And when I spoke to a German colleague who had moved to the Netherlands just recently, he told me that in the large university hospital where he had worked in Germany, until eight years ago, caesarian sections were still being carried out under a general anaesthetic because they were "afraid of the consequences of using a regional technique". There was in the 1980s a second reason why some German colleagues chose to give a general anaesthetic for Caesarian section. The act of placing a tube in the airway could be billed whereas an epidural anaesthetic could not. Effectively this created an incentive to ignore the science and follow the money.

Doctor's decisions are guided far more by emotion than they would like to admit.

Studies are essential, and difficult

There are important ethical considerations before setting up a trial. For instance, let us suppose that there is a drug used against a certain cancer, and strong reasons to believe it is effective, but no statistical proof. It would not be ethical to carry out a study in which half the patients were given a placebo to create a control group because it would be reasonable to believe that they would have less chance of surviving. If in the same situation two drugs are being used, both believed to be more or less equally effective, then it would be ethical and useful to compare the results of both drugs, to see which is best. This is why it is mandatory to have trials evaluated by an independent ethical committee before they may be started.

One simple example of how trials have changed things for the better is arthroscopy of the knee, in which an instrument is introduced into the knee joint, so that it can be visualised and treated if necessary. In my time this was a real money spinner for the industry supplying the apparatus and disposable material, and the surgeons did quite well out of it too. But when studies were carried out comparing arthroscopic surgery with no surgery, the conclusion was unavoidable: looking at both groups of patients a year later showed that there was very little difference in symptoms and disability. It was clear that surgeons had being carrying out an enormous number of operations all over the world, with very little to show for it. Medical research of this sort encourages doctors to abandon useless procedures, and refine their indications for an operation. In this way, the number of arthroscopies being carried out in developed countries such as the Netherlands has dropped drastically leaving a much smaller   group for which such surgery seems appropriate.

It is interesting to take a step back and look at how such a situation comes to exist. It is not a coincidence that many surgeons are in private practice, and get payed per operation. So, if you have a patient in front of you, and you think, "I could suggest waiting a year to see how it goes, or I could carry out an operation." Both approaches would have been quite acceptable before the statistics came out. So it is not surprising that a doctor who had just bought a second house in France might (consciously or unconsciously) choose the operative procedure. And doctors are always egged on by the industry that stands to earn massive amounts of money from these operations. So the industry arranges seminars, and sends doctors on trips to a ski area, where they may learn about the newest techniques (and perhaps do a bit of skiing??). The doctors who carry out the largest number of operations are considered to be experts, and asked to talk at such meetings. As you may imagine, they do not usually stand up and say that it is all a giant waste of money and manpower, not to mention the complications always inherent in surgery.

It is only fair to point out that doctors in such situations are usually genuinely convinced that they are working in the best interests of the patients. For more on this, see the chapter on cognitive dissonance. One of the disadvantages of private practice is that there is a financial incentive involved in medical choices. This is one of the reasons that I preferred hospital service. I shall certainly have earned far less than I could have, but it has always been more important to me not to have financial factors driving my professional choices.

The fact is that studies are a mixed blessing. In the arthroscopy example the studies lead to an important change in medical care, and a reduction in costs to the health insurers, and complications for the patient. Fortunately this is more and more the case, but even when studies are carried out, they may be flawed, for different reasons.

Research - what goes wrong

Unfortunately there are also frauds in the medical community. Cases have come to light in which some or all of the data was fabricated by the doctor carrying out the study. The results led to patients being given wrong diagnoses and wrong treatments. There have been many high-profile examples of such fraud with very serious consequences for patients.

A doctor carrying out a study is not only looking for the truth. Usually the ego is also at work, wanting to elevate the professional profile, perhaps leading to the position of professor or an expert who is looked up to. The doctor is under pressure from the industry, which is often paying for the study, and wants a positive outcome for their shareholders. It is not unusual for companies to block publication of unfavourable papers; the doctor feels these double pressures, and the incentive is there for him to "bend" his results to suit the case. It is easy to do — drop a few patients out of a study, and the statistics are suddenly on your side, as it were.

The pharmaceutical industry has a particularly bad record in this respect, and million dollar fines have been frequent in the past years, as the industry massages the results, and the doctors, to promote a drug or treatment which is ineffective or downright dangerous.

One particularly pernicious example is the PSA test for prostate cancer. I shall not go into the details, but this test has caused endless suffering, and almost certainly deaths, as it leads to unnecessary surgery causing serious complications and does not improve the survival rate among patients at all. As a result of very hard fought battles, and some good studies which reversed the findings of previous studies, the PSA test is now being used more on indication than as a population screening. It is a prime example of the industry and the involved doctors running amok, often making fortunes over the backs of the patients.

If the reader wishes more information on such matters, then the book "Bad Pharma" by Ben Goldacre is a good, if shocking, place to start. "The Great Prostate Hoax" by Richard Ablin and Ronald Piana, about the PSA test is also a very revealing and disturbing read. Ablin developed the PSA test, and is disgusted with how it has been misused.

When to believe the results.

In the light of the above, it becomes relevant to know when to believe the results of a study. It is possible to write a very convincing article which can be torn to shreds by a statistician. So we need to look at a number of factors that may lead us to consider the results to be reliable.

1: Who funded the research? As soon as financial support is involved from a company that stands to gain from the conclusion reached, we should be extra careful. The conclusions may be fine, but manipulation is frequent.

2: Has the article been reviewed by experts in the field before publication?

3: Have the findings been replicated in another study from another group? It is a sad fact that only a small percentage of medical studies have been successfully replicated.

Consider the situation in social psychology. There have been very many research studies which have been carried out with the serious intent to produce valid results, but which have since been dismissed for a variety of reasons — bad methodology, misuse of statistics, too small numbers of participants, etc. Sometimes it can get very personal, sometimes based on factors such as jealousy and then the truth gets tied up in a whole mess of claims, derogatory remarks, and counter-claims. Careers can be broken. The furore over Amy Cuddy's work on "power poses" and their effects on self-confidence is a classic example.

Take home message

The fact that a treatment has not been proved to be effective does not mean that it is not effective. It may just be that no study has been carried out, and it could also be that a study has been carried out and come to incorrect conclusions. Inversely, the fact that a treatment has been demonstrated to be effective by a medical trial does not necessarily mean that it is effective. It may also be the result of a bad trial design, or deliberate manipulation of the trial data. It's complicated.

Despite this rather negative chapter, without trials, we should still be living in a world of treatment only dictated by beliefs and misconceptions. There is much to improve, but good research is absolutely fundamental to progress in the medical field.

To be happy for an hour, get drunk;
to be happy for a year, fall in love;
to be happy for the rest of your life;
take up gardening

Chinese proverb

Dealing with patient dissatisfaction

I use the word dissatisfaction and not complaints deliberately. A doctor who deals adequately with dissatisfaction will rarely be confronted with an official complaint.

I heard of one woman who took her two year old boy to the casualty unit many years ago. He had been playing with her purse, put a coin into his mouth and choked on it. On arrival in the hospital he was a grey-blue colour and his breathing was just audible. He hung like a rag doll in his mother's arms. The ENT specialist rushed with him to the operating theatre, and performed an emergency laryngoscopy without any anaesthetic; the child was unconscious anyway. He extracted a shilling coin, and the child recovered within minutes with only oxygen being given. The doctor went to the mother and said, "Madam, you brought him just in time: another five minutes and he would have been dead. He's fine now, and here is the shilling piece he swallowed." The mother reacted with fury: she shouted, "It was a two shilling piece he swallowed, and I want it back".

Presumably she had visions of the doctor sneaking out of the back door, and blowing the money on a bag of chips. Some patients can draw blood from under your nails!

One difficulty in talking to patients about complications, is that they nearly always have difficulty distinguishing, "It went badly" from "It was done badly". I shall try to explain the difference with an example. If you were on the intensive care department, and you had no known allergies, it is still possible that you would have a life threatening allergic reaction to an antibiotic I gave you. It <u>went</u> badly; this is a complication, not a medical error. If you had <u>warned</u> me that you were allergic and I forgot, and gave you the drug anyway, then I <u>did</u> it badly, and this is a medical error. Even then many patients and their families just don't seem to <u>want</u> to understand the differ-

103

ence. Emotionally they seem to need someone to blame, someone to vent their anger on.

If a tree falls on your car in a storm, there is no one to be angry at. Unless you are able to say, "The neighbours should have cut that tree down years ago — they knew it was rotten". This would be much more satisfying; we have a need to vent.

I once had a patient who developed a thrombosis in one of the arteries leading to his spinal cord. It caused what is called an anterior spinal artery syndrome, and he never walked again. To make things worse, I had given him an epidural anaesthetic. Try to imagine how hard it was to go to him and say, "I'm so sorry you're paralysed, and I know I stuck a needle in your back, but I did nothing wrong". Well, would _you_ believe that? And yet it was the truth. I spoke a lot to that man and his family, and they never made a complaint. But each meeting was agonising because I could not admit to the mistake they were sure I'd made. Even knowing that I did nothing wrong, such cases as this one will remain with me until I die.

You need a certain amount of toughness and to have your empathy under control to deal with such events without going under yourself. It is however an example of how, even with such a disastrous complication, it is possible to prevent an official complaint by showing a family that you care, and that what has happened is deeply painful to yourself. They probably thought that I was covering up, but I think they liked me, and they let it be.

It sounds so counter-intuitive, but I genuinely believe that it would have been far easier to have made an error, and been able to admit to it. Then they would have believed me immediately, and found it easier to forgive me. And I am afraid that I have an example of that to prove it.

A sixteen year old girl came for an operation on her vocal cords. Normally we gave a general anaesthetic through a tube we introduced through the vocal cords, but that makes it hard for the ENT surgeon to get a good view of the cords. In such cases we had a special tube which sat below the larynx, and was held in place by a balloon or cuff that pressed on the side wall of the airway. There were two very thin tubes passing into this through the cords, one to inflate the cuff, and one to administer oxygen under pressure to the lungs. Don't ask me how, but I managed to connect the high pressure to the cuff inflating tube; and inflate it did, exploding with a loud bang. I felt over her windpipe, and could feel air under the skin (it's compared to feeling eggshells crackling). I wanted to disappear through the floor. We ended the procedure, and took the girl to the intensive care department. I then had the daunting task of approaching the parents to tell them what I had done, and I did so transparently. I must have looked so incredibly miserable that they were very understanding, and seemed almost more concerned for me than their daughter. I am happy to report that this incident lead to no permanent damage, and the girl went home next day. Such incidents make one realise that we are walking such a thin line between success and disaster with each patient.

In an earlier chapter, I described how an air traffic accident would automatically lead to an investigation, and the results would be shared world-wide, to warn others, and make necessary changes to avoid repetition. In the above mentioned case we adapted the equipment to make repetition impossible, but that was just in our own hospital. At that time we did not even pause to think about disseminating this information to help others. It seems so obvious in retrospect.

As long as humans are running the show, mistakes will be made, and I have made my share of them. Nevertheless I should like to point out at this juncture that I <u>have</u> had patients survive my anaesthetics from time to time, but that would fit in a chapter over patient *satisfaction*, which is probably unnecessary.

When having a meeting with a dissatisfied patient, your most powerful tool is listening. Your biggest enemy is defensiveness. Take your time to listen to the patient's story. Try to put yourself into their shoes, and look at the situation through their eyes. How would you feel if it had happened to you? Ask questions to clarify. Ask what effect the complication is having on their lives. Remember, patients who complain want, above all else, to be heard.

If you have done something wrong, say you are sorry, and that you will use the situation to learn. If you have done nothing wrong, say something like, "I'm so sorry this has happened to you." This is not an admission, it is a demonstration of empathy. An example:

When we perform nerve blocks with patients, occasionally a patient may have minor nerve dysfunction, even when the procedure has been carried out perfectly. Of these, about ninety-nine percent recover spontaneously in time. If you are the one that doesn't, then you may have a real problem. Here it is a question of, "I'm sorry this happened to you" and not "I messed up".

Patients need to be informed of possible complications, and these days to sign an "informed consent" form. The difficulty is, deciding where to draw the line. Do I really need to inform patients that there is a chance that they will wake up under the anaesthetic and during the operation? This is very rare, but it does happen, and it is very traumatic when it does. For me the most important question is, "Does this information help the patient to make an informed decision about treatment?"

A patient coming for a cosmetic operation should probably be given more information, as they have the choice to cancel the operation if they do not want to run the risks involved. But when an operation is vital, and needs to be carried out under a general anaesthetic then you are really not helping the patient by informing them that they might wake up during the operation. You are achieving two other things — protecting yourself from liability, and frightening the patient. I have always tried to walk the narrow path between telling a patient what they need to know without frightening them unnecessarily; my own liability comes in third place.

There is also a medico-legal side to this; certainly in the past, medical insurers have advised doctors very strongly never to admit responsibility when something goes wrong. Of course that is in their interest, but it is not necessarily in your interest, or that of the patient or family. It is certainly something to keep in mind when dealing with such situations. If there is any doubt about culpability, then it is better to tell the patient that this will be investigated, and that they will be informed of the results. That is fair to all parties. If there is no doubt, honesty is the best policy.

Take-home message

People are so forgiving if they know you are being honest. They don't expect you to be perfect, but they do expect you to be truthful. Tell them what happened, tell them how you feel, and tell them that you would support an official complaint when you mess up, and it will rarely get that far.

The doctor gives the tablet, and with the tablet he gives the word. Without the word the tablet doesn't work.

Chinese saying

From the humble placebo to body language

Mind over body

I have often stood by a nurse giving an antiemetic and said with surprise, "Are you allowed to give that stuff without a special order? It's good, but it's incredibly expensive". Ignoring the ethics for a moment, I think you then give a more effective drug.

The placebo effect occurs when a treatment, which has in itself no beneficial effect on body or mind, causes a positive physiological or psychological effect as a result of the expectations the patient has. The effects are produced by the patient himself, largely unconsciously; although strangely enough, in some studies patients were told that they were being given a placebo and it was still effective.

The placebo is generally greatly underrated, and often spoken of with derision. It conjures up an image of a dusty doctor giving a sugar coated pill to a patient. But the placebo is far, far more than this. It is probably safe to say that there is no medical treatment without some element of the placebo effect. The effect of a drug may be influenced simply by the way it is given. These effects can go surprisingly far. In some placebo controlled trials of painkillers, it has proven difficult to distinguish between the analgesic effect of morphine and a placebo.

If someone is given a dummy morphine injection, and knows which side effects are possible, then these effects, such as nausea, may be experienced next to the beneficial effects. Instead of a placebo, we then have a nocibo.

109

Even more interesting to me are two studies of the relapse rate after treatment of an ulcer (one in Germany and one in Denmark). The surprising finding was that relapse was five times more common in the groups receiving the effective treatment than the ones with a placebo. I have a theory as to what could be behind this very unexpected phenomenon: if, after the trial has ended, your brain learns that the healing was its own work, then it realises that it has the power to treat the condition without external drugs. If it believes that healing was dependent on an external factor, then it is primed to think that without that factor, the ulcer may come back.

We know that our minds are programmed to attach more credit to information when a number of conditions are met. One is high status; this is why doctors, and even better professors, feature so often in advertising. A placebo pill given by a doctor will work better than one given by your neighbour, but not as well as one prescribed by a professor.

We know that a blue pill works better as a tranquilliser, and a red one as a painkiller; it has to do with expectations and associations within the brain.

If you find this unconvincing, then maybe one of Derren Brown's programmes might change your mind. (Derren Brown - Fear and faith). In it, he showed how the placebo effect could be introduced and strengthened by adding layers of believability. He took a number of volunteers and told them of a drug which could eliminate the fear response. The story was that it was developed for the military, and was now being introduced to the public. The volunteers were taken to a laboratory which was in fact only a mock-up. There they had a talk from one of the 'researchers' who had developed this drug, and they were shown a video about it.

The effects were little short of dramatic. One man, who had such a fear of heights that even crossing a little bridge over a stream made him anxious, ended upon the parapet of a high bridge with no fear at all. At that point Brown told him that it was just a placebo pill. The subject was unfazed; he had lost his fear of heights, and the fact that he had produced this effect without a pill was probably just a plus.

In the meantime it has been shown that the placebo can work not only for phobias, but also for allergies and eczema. What it comes down to, is that our minds are clearly able to influence our bodily reactions to a surprising extent, and that there is more than one way to illicit this effect.

This is all tied up with the well known fact that if you believe something, you tend to make it become true. A disturbing example of this was the study carried out in America, in which teachers were told that the children in their class were either gifted, or were low performers. In fact there was no real difference between the groups. The interesting and worrying thing is that the children came to live up (or down) to the teacher's expectation. The "gifted" group outperformed the group described as low performers.

Tell a child that he is no good at drawing, and you have sown a belief which may prevent the child from ever being a good artist. Beware the beliefs you put into the receptive mind of a child! I think that this is closely related to the placebo effect: tell your mind that a sugar pill will give pain relief, and the brain causes the necessary outpouring of endogenous opiates to make it come true. Tell your mind that you are no good at something, and your mind will make sure that your behaviour fits your belief.

One practical situation where we doctors should certainly take account of this effect is in our daily contacts with patients. It seems certain that our own expectations will influence the patient, and that an optimistic doctor will produce, in general, better results than a pessimistic one. Our optimism is a placebo, our pessimism a nocebo. This underlines the truth of the old saying at the beginning of this chapter: the doctor gives the tablet, and with the tablet he gives the word.....

This may all sound very fuzzy, but it is quite clear that our brains have some peculiar habits which would cause Mr. Spock from Startrek to raise an amused eyebrow.

The placebo reaction works stronger for some people than for others and depends partly on the "suggestibility" of a person, and I would guess that the same people will also be susceptible to hypnosis. This trait is often

111

equated with weakness, but that is far too simple an explanation. It is diffi-cult to hypnotise people with a very low IQ. Some people seem to be able to create very vivid and convincing mental constructs, of which images are the most common. It may perhaps just as well be seen as a strength rather than as a weakness; although suggestibility can make you vulnerable, it can also be a great help in some situations.

The whole question of placebos is tightly connected with the relatively new science of psycho-neuro-immunology. This considers ways in which our thoughts, neurological systems and immune systems are intimately connect-ed. A very interesting and readable book on research into the subject is "The Balance Within" by Esther Sternberg.

Body over mind

The mind body interaction is powerful and works in both directions. Our thoughts and expectations can influence physiological processes. Changing body language can influence how we feel. This much is certain. There is much uncertainty as to how far this effect goes; my guess is that for some patients it goes very far, and for some it may not work at all. The terms "placebo responders" and "non-responders" describes this phenomenon, but that suggests an all or nothing response, which it clearly is not.

Many people hate public speaking, and feel dreadfully uncertain when they have to do so. The same goes for interviews. Both groups could do well to watch confident people, and just model their body language. Using this 'language' the next time they talk or sit in a job interview will make them feel more confident, and people who project self confidence are judged to be so. "Fake it till you make it" is the idea. In its most simple form, people who are uncertain have a closed posture and make themselves small, people who are confident have an open posture and make themselves look larger. This is very important in interview situations, where coming over as confi-dent will greatly increase your chances. Scientific studies to demonstrate this effect have been carried out, and some support the idea. The studies them-selves have come in for criticism, but my personal experience convinces me that there is much truth to the idea.

112

A eureka moment for me was when I was working for a couple of weeks in Kenya's university hospital. I can remember walking up a broad flight of stairs, with a busy stream of families, doctors and nurses going up and down. I realised all at once that I was dodging left and right to avoid other people, and asked myself why I was the one continually doing the avoiding. I came to the conclusion that it had to do with my self-image, or sense of self-worth. The next day I visualised my image as large, bright and confident, and walked straight up-stairs, and others moved to avoid me. It was for me a rather strange and exciting experience — the realisation came to me that my self-image does not have to be fixed, and that when I change it, then others perceive and react to me differently.

Take-home message

Our brains can have a powerful influence on our bodies and vice versa. Usually this is unconscious, but it is also possible to make use of these effects consciously. Do not underestimate what these processes can mean to yourself and your patients.

If you want a quality, act as if you already had it. Try the "as if" technique.

William james

The fragility of reputation

R eputations can be created and destroyed in seconds. And your reputation has to do with more than just the facts of the case. My wife's
nieces are staying with us for the weekend, and it reminds me of the
last time they were here. They were about two and four years old, and when
they saw me in my dressing gown, the older child pointed with amazement
and said, "Uncle Nigel's wearing a dress". She had never seen a man in a
dressing gown before. When they left, I said to my wife that I was glad that
they live in a different town. I could just imagine the little girl visiting a
friend and telling her in the presence of her parents what she had seen. In
no time it would be general knowledge that a transvestite lives in that little
farmhouse... "An 'im a doctor an' all!"

Francesco Schettino, captain of the Costa Concordia, was at one moment
the most prestigious and powerful man on the large cruise ship, standing on
the bridge with a lady friend. He was going to perform a close sail-past of
an island. Minutes later the ship was on the rocks, and he was allegedly one
of the first to leave the sinking ship. Just a few minutes work, and although
there may well have been extenuating circumstances, he was put in prison,
his reputation in tatters.

Recently Dominique Strauss-Kahn, one time head of the International
Monetary Fund, one of the most powerful people in the world, and at one
time possible future president of France was facing a trial for sexual mis-
demeanours. The matter was later resolved for an undisclosed amount. But
he has thrown away a glittering career. How the mighty are fallen!

Coming closer to home, scientists, medical or otherwise, regularly ruin a
good reputation simply by so desperately needing a better one that they

make claims based on falsified data which lift them close to the stars before crashing onto the rocks of reality when the truth is revealed.

Hwang Woo-Sun is a south Korean scientist who was a rising star in the field of cloning. There were those who expected him to get a Nobel prize for his discovery of a way to produce human embryonic stem cells. Then his work turned out to be fraudulent, and his reputation was shattered. This is no rare occurrence, and in many cases the scientists concerned were genuine high flyers in their own area.

This burning desire for fame, which is so common, and which undermines the reputation of medical science itself, must have its roots in some underlying psychological flaw — in the doctor's ego. I would guess it comes down to low self-esteem.

Some people have what is called an external locus of control; they see their lives as controlled by factors outside themselves. They tend to see themselves as at the mercy of influences from without. When things go wrong, it is always the result of other people and forces outside their control. Their destiny is shaped for them. They often have a sense of powerlessness. If asked how they know when they have done well, they will typically react by saying that they got praise from other people.

People with an internal locus of control have far more the idea that they are the masters of their own destiny; their sense of worth is internal, and less dependent on what others think. If asked how they know when they have done well, they will typically react by saying that they have an inner sense of when they perform well, and look to the results achieved.

A perfect example of this was described by the American coach and author Anthony Robbins. It is the case of two brothers, born into a family where father was a criminal and alcoholic. One followed in his father's footsteps the other became CEO of a large company. When asked how they came to be where they were, the first answered, "What do you expect with such a father as example" the other said, "having seen the example of my father, I determined that I was going to do it differently." Same circumstances, one internal and one external locus of control. It's not so much what happens to us, but how we process that internally.

One major difference between these two types is in empowerment. Knowing that the cause of things going right or wrong lies outside yourself implies that you are fairly powerless to bring change. Knowing that the source of your happiness and achievements is in yourself puts you in the driving seat, as it were. It is empowering.

Part of this difference may be genetic, but I am sure that it is the early years of life which decide. The presence or absence of unconditional love in these early years has a tremendous and largely unrecognised influence. In her brilliant book, "Why love matters," the British psychiatrist Sue Gerhardt demonstrates the psychological and physiological consequences of the presence or absence of love in the formative years. And the consequences are huge.

I would love to see a study in which the childhood years of scientists who get onto the wrong path are compared to those who do not succumb to such temptation. Such a study might not be so easy due to the possible presence of a group who's dishonesty just never got found out! I believe that Alfred Mendel, father of genetics, was not above manipulating his data. He was lucky that his hunch paid off.

In the above cases their reputations were broken by their own dealings. That is not always the case. At the time of writing Pakistan has a blasphemy law. Any person who insults a religion or deity or, in most cases, Mohammed may be liable to a long prison sentence or even a death sentence. There are politicians in that country who wanted to change this law. In some cases they have been murdered for it. Many of the people accused of blasphemy have also been killed before they could even come to trial. The level of evidence needed to be found guilty is low: hearsay is enough. In one recent instance a Christian woman had a row with two Muslim women. After this incident the two accused her of blasphemy against the prophet. There were no other witnesses nor any proof, but in the meantime the Christian woman and her family have been driven out of their village, and someone else has taken over her house. She is still alive at the time of writing, but I imagine that she fears for her life. At the end of the story there is a life and a reputation ruined; quite possibly simply because the other two women wanted to hurt her.

There are people who say that they don't care a damn what others think of them. Well, such people probably exist, but I would guess they are rare, and that beneath the surface they do care a damn. I think that we are genetically programmed to care about our reputation. It's part of being members of a 'tribe'. Our position in the pecking order is partly dependent on the way others think about us. Our chances of happy relationships and a successful career are greatly influenced by the opinion others have of us.

We form impressions of other people extremely quickly, and very often accurately. After that we have a strong inbuilt tendency to maintain that first impression. We notice everything that supports our judgement, and are blind to information which might change it. This is called "confirmation bias".

Let me give an example: I work for the first time with a new surgeon, and for the first three operations he causes a lot of blood loss. This could just be bad luck; it happens to the best, but my first impression is that this is not a very careful surgeon. I tell my colleagues, and this impression starts to spread. After that, we all notice any cases with blood-loss, and don't notice the cases with little loss. This surgeon is going to have a hard time convincing us that we might just have formed an unfair impression.

This may be a bit of a caricature, but the underlying truth is clear enough: "First impressions matter" is simply a statement of fact. This is why in job interviews it is very important to show yourself as confident and likeable. Don't underestimate that likeable bit. We want to help people we like, and we want to have people we like around us. If two applicants for a job have exactly the same qualifications, then the one who comes in with a friendly smile will probably be chosen.

First impressions are important for a second reason, and that is the 'halo' effect. Most people have never even heard of this, and yet we are all influenced by it. If we rate someone highly for one reason, then we tend to rate them higher in other areas where it may or may not be deserved. If you think that someone is a brilliant surgeon, there is a tendency to think that he or she is a better driver or cook without looking for supporting evidence. Our first impression is followed by a halo of respect, as it were. Of course the opposite is also true; a bad first impression leads to a negative halo. You can be on the giving or the receiving end of this.

Take home messages

First impressions do count, and while we are generally amazingly accurate in our intuitive judgements, when we get it wrong, it can lead to misunderstandings and problems. Keep the threshold low for changing your opinions, and beware the halo effect!

Setting a high standard for yourself is valuable to you, and to all around you. Valuing your reputation above integrity is where it all starts to fall apart.

People are always blaming their circumstances for what they are.

I don't believe in circumstances.

The people who get on in this world are the people who get up and look for the circumstances they want, and, if they can't find them, make them.

George Bernard Shaw

In search of happiness

To some extent people seem to have a built in thermostat for happiness. Some are by nature more somber and others more cheerful. This thermostat seems to be fairly constant over long time periods and to some extent independent of external factors. Some studies have shown that people who's circumstances have deteriorated seriously — for instance after coming hemiplegic in a car accident — eventually rate themselves as happy as they were in the past.

That said, there is no doubt that our happiness is influenced by how we think, and in thinking we use words and images. The words we use have a tremendous effect on how we feel, and most people are unaware of this. If you arrive at work and say, "The traffic was horrific, and I was almost too late at work," this will produce a slightly different feeling than when you say, "there was heavy traffic, and I still managed to get to work on time". Insignificant difference, I hear you say, but multiply this difference by all the things you say in a day and you can be in a completely different state of mind by the time you arrive back home. This is why the choice of words you use to think and to speak is so important. Change "he is quite impossible to work with" into, "he is a challenge to work with" and you have in a subtle way started to change the relationship.

If you are doing a job you don't like, look first to see whether you can change your approach so that you do enjoy your work. For instance, take on some extra tasks which you do enjoy, or find ways to influence the activity or working atmosphere to one you like. And if you can't, then it's time to think of changing your job. We spend far too much of our lives at work to be doing something that does not make us happy. (Reading this back, I realise that, whilst I believe that what I have written is generally true, there are millions of people around the world who have no choice, and who are doing dirty, unhealthy, backbreaking jobs for whom the ideas of this paragraph may seem a cruel joke.)

Diverging slightly from the main subject here, it is interesting to look at how different religious and non-religious people are in how they live their lives. If you ask both, "What is the meaning of life?" you will get a quite different answer. I am an atheist, and my answer will be simple: "there is no inherent meaning to life". This sounds pretty dismal, but it doesn't have to be. I can create my own meaning, and my own goals. My main goal is to enjoy life as much as possible without hurting others. I don't busy myself with thoughts of the afterlife; when I'm dead I'm gone.

Whereas the meaning of my life is an internal creation, for religious people, the meaning comes from outside. First you have to believe in a god, and then, through the ages, words of meaning are put into his mouth, as it were, and that is then the meaning of life.

So what makes someone happy? It may seem counterintuitive, but, if you leave the religious trappings aside, it may be hard to tell by behaviour alone whether someone is or is not religious. Things that are "good" in the biblical sense, are also often the things that make us happy. This is no coincidence; we are hard-wired to get a reward (feelings of happiness) when we behave in ways which are important to the survival of ourselves and our group. Most religions emphasise such behaviour. Unfortunately, as the centuries pass, they tend to add a lot of stuff which messes the whole thing up, and has been the cause of endless strife and misery. Not withstanding this, regular churchgoers have been shown to be happier and less depressed than non-churchgoers. This may well be due to the community spirit and sense of mutual support.

However, careful analysis of the external behaviour of believers suggests that they are no more likely to demonstrate religious values in their behaviour toward others than non-believers are.

We know that amassing a great fortune or vast amounts of material goods does not make us any happier in the long run. A certain amount of material comfort is necessary to be happy, but the increase in happiness tails off once the basic needs of life have been met. I shall never forget the young man who guided me to my island paradise on Lake Malawi. He radiated happiness, and probably had almost nothing. I asked him if he had plans, and he said that he wanted to set up a hotel. I did not say it, but I could not help thinking of all the overweight businessmen I had seen in the capital city driving around in their expensive cars, and looking miserable. I hoped this young man would not follow that path. One reason really rich people are generally not happier than the general population is because it has een shown that they look less to what they have and more to comparing their wealth to that of others. There will always be people with more, which is a bron of dissatisfaction. There will be exceptions to this, and my guess would be that the exceptions are the rich people who are also philan-thropists. They are more focussed on the good they can do with their wealth and less with their position on the ladder.

In the meantime a great deal of study has gone into what makes us happy. The top two are perhaps helping others and getting into the flow. The first needs no explanation, although it does raise questions about what egotism is. If we give to others and feel good as a result, is that being egotistical? Is that even a relevant question? It is not hard to look around and find "givers" and "takers" in life, and then it is fairly obvious which are the hap-pier. So whether it is at work or outside it, helping others is one way of making life more enjoyable for yourself.

Getting into the flow is another matter. It means doing something you like to do, and getting lost in it. In this state nothing exists outside of what you are doing. The poet lost in composition, the child losing itself building a sand-castle, the musician aware only of the music; suddenly you come back down to earth and discover that hours have flown by without you noticing. For more about this I can recommend the book, "Finding Flow," by Mihaly Csikszentmihalyi.

This has been a long digression, but I come back to the last chapter; when I am at work I want to enjoy myself, to be at play more than at work. If I engage with others, whether it be patient or co-worker, in such a way that they feel good, then at the end of the day I shall feel a happier person for it.

I want to give my co-workers the following feelings: that I hear them, that I respect them, that I need them.

For patients it is: I hear you, and appreciate your concerns, I make jokes, so it can't be a big deal, and at the same time I am on top of the ball, and you're in good hands.

(Sometimes we know that there are better hands than ours; we have to live with that thought, but the patient doesn't. On some occasions we can call in those better hands to help (if we can climb over our egos)! When I worked as a junior doctor in Zambia, my patients were in terribly inexperienced and half-competent hands, but there <u>was</u> no one else. It would not have helped them to know of my shortcomings, so I put on a brave face.)

Talking of jokes brings me to another point. For good reason it is said that laughter is the best medicine. There is much truth in that. Laughing makes us and others feel better and it lowers the levels of stress hormones. I know that during medical meetings, my use of humor often broke tensions, making agreement easier. It has been shown convincingly that just putting on a smile makes us feel happier. Many schools of meditation advise students to put on a slight smile while meditating. It's not a coincidence that many Buddha figures show a slight smile. Just walking through the corridors giving people a big smile will make you feel better, and you will be surprised how many smiles you get in return. It may feel strange at first, but just observe how people react, and how it makes you feel. Like so many things in this book, I suggest you give it a try, and hold on to those things that work for you and drop those that don't.

Take home message

Although achieving happiness is not completely within our control, there are a number of relatively simple strategies which can certainly help in that direction.

Happiness?
A good cigar, a good meal,
And a good woman
Or a bad woman.
It depends on how much happiness
you can handle.

George Burns

Mindfulness & Meditation

Mindfulness is one of those subjects that often tend to be thought of as 'airy-fairy'. We medical people tend to pride ourselves on our scientific thinking and decision making. Things like mindfulness and meditation tend not to fit in with the way we see the world. We would, however, do well to be a little more humble. After all, what is 'scientific'? To most of us it implies that we base our treatments on clinically proven theories. What we tend to forget is that what is clinically proven today may be completely debunked tomorrow. The examples are legio.

Thirty years ago it became clear on the basis of clinical studies that eating fats was bad for us, and the main cause of cardiovascular diseases. At that time there was an English professor, John Yudkin, who maintained that it was not the fats that were doing the damage as much as sugar. He wrote a book called, "Pure, white and deadly" in which he set out his arguments. He was made a laughing stock by the American researcher who claimed that fat was the problem, and the food industry, especially the sugar manufactures, fell over themselves to undermine his authority and arguments. The food industry was having a wonderful time producing 'light' products which were held to be more healthy, and were certainly much more expensive. Eating butter was considered by them to be life threatening.

In the meantime, we have learned that the science was faulty, and that Yudkin was right. The sugar industry is still in denial, but gradually sugar is being phased out of food and drinks, and butter is being rehabilitated.

Yes, the science was faulty. And science is faulty partly due to the egos of the scientists and doctors involved (see the chapter on reputation), and partly due to attaching importance to studies which were in themselves faulty. It is generally agreed that something is only scientifically proven when the results of a study are replicated by other researchers. But the disconcerting fact is that only a small percentage of medical studies have actually been replicated. This is fairly shocking, and there are at least two reasons for it: researchers prefer to do new research above replicating old studies. New research is where the Nobel prizes lie. The second reason is that medical journals are heavily tilted toward new research, and especially toward research with positive findings. This means that even if a scientist repeats a study, the chances of it being published are small and even smaller if it discounts the original positive outcomes.

Why this digression? What I want to illustrate is that things that have been scientifically proven are not necessarily true, and things that have not been proven by science are not necessarily false. We need to be more subtle when forming judgements about what is good for our patients, and what is good for ourselves. In general I think it fair to say that ideas that have been shown time and again to be true deserve more credence than the results of one or two studies (scepticism should be multiplied tenfold when commercial producers of medicines and apparatus are involved in the studies). So now we are getting back to the point.

I stand firmly on the side of those who claim that mindfulness would be of great and practical value to all of us. There have been many studies over the years that suggest that mindfulness and meditation have a powerful positive influence on mind and body. The power of the mind to influence bodily functions and vice versa is continually becoming clearer. I know of no studies suggesting that mindfulness has any negative effects. There have been cases recorded of people who have experienced psychological problems during mindfulness meditation, but these are probably people with serious problems, which have been suppressed and which come to the surface during meditation. If people become uncomfortable during mindfulness, then that is a sign that they would do well to look for psychological support. Yoga has not without reason stressed the importance of expert guidance during meditation. Problems caused by meditation seem to be extremely rare, whereas the vast majority of people will benefit.

I write in the Trump era, in which people are being blasted with negative thoughts at an unprecedented rate. Psychiatrists in America recognise the "Trump effect". There is an increase in people with anxiety disorders, and psychic traumas which seem to be "revitalised" by the confusion, anger, and polarisation this president brings with him. For half of America this is a president who can do nothing wrong, whilst the other half experience chronic anxiety at the thought of this man having unfettered access to America's nuclear weapons. Just in such a time it is so important for people to be able to tune out all this noise, and experience the calm that comes with mindfulness or meditation.

Mindfulness and meditation have been shown to influence a wide variety of mental and physical functions, causing positive mood, less depression, improved powers of concentration, lower blood pressure and a stronger immune system. There is even evidence that cell telomeres are longer in expert meditators, and these are one of the markers of longevity.

Mindfulness and meditation are not the same thing. Mindfulness implies being intensely aware of what we are doing in the present moment. So if I am gardening and am completely focused on feeling the earth between my fingers, seeing, feeling and smelling a flower, and hearing the sounds around me with nothing else on my mind, then that is mindfulness. If I am gardening and listening to a podcast at the same time, that is not. Meditation is more ambitious, and harder. It comes down to narrowing the focus of attention to a single point, at which time one is thinking of nothing. Various tools are used to achieve this state, such as mantras and concentration on breathing. Most people find it intensely difficult to achieve a blank mind. So, in a nutshell, mindfulness is for everyone, meditation is for the few who are prepared to take on the really hard work.

Only recently a study on children aged nine to eleven in schools in Canada showed fairly dramatic improvements in a number of parameters of behaviour and arithmetic when a programme including mindfulness was given over a period of a few months.

I wonder why it is that so many people who pride themselves on their intellectual prowess and will readily accept the results of a single scientific study of a surgical technique still completely reject the idea that mindfulness might well be better for us than a whole cupboard full of medical potions and tablets. And I don't have a good answer to that question. It is true that some disciplines, such as psycho-neuro-immunology, are still young, and perhaps not so well known. But the positive effects of meditation and mindfulness have been known for centuries.

In the face of the known evidence, it is curious, to say the least, that very, very few people I have known apply meditation or mindfulness seriously in their daily lives. I can think of a number of reasons: a conservative and blinkered look on life, the pace of modern life, modern communication technology, laziness and disillusion.

The first and second are probably linked. A natural tendency to stay with what we know and what is 'normal,' exacerbated by the fact that we are all so busy, and have very little time for such esoteric matters. You may say with some justification, "It's all right for you to be so self righteous, you are retired, and have all the time in the world. We didn't hear so much from you when you had a full time job, and children, and a house and garden….."

It is true that the pace of modern life makes it much harder to find the time to meditate. On the other hand, there is good reason to believe that time spent on meditation can be seen as an investment. By clearing the mind and recharging the batteries, there is an increase in efficiency which probably more than compensates the time spent meditating.

Modern communication means that we are bombarded with information from the moment we wake until we go to sleep (and afterward if we are not careful). E-mail, instant messaging, Facebook, online news, gaming, etc. What most people don't stop to realise is that all these things use up mental energy, and that is a finite resource. We are almost constantly so called 'multitasking'; driving and using the telephone, eating and reading, talking with the t.v. on. However, we only think that we are multitasking, because in fact what we are doing is rapidly switching back and forth between tasks, with a resultant drop in effectiveness in both tasks. Who in these times eats a meal, and only thinks about what he is eating? I think that mindfulness and meditation have always been valuable, and that they are only becoming more essential as the demands made on our brains continue to grow.

Laziness was the last reason I mentioned why meditation gets pushed aside. It's really difficult, and demands more self-discipline than most people are prepared to exercise. There is also no immediate result to keep up motivation. In this, I must look first to myself. I believe implicitly in its value, and yet I do precious little about it. I sit for ten minutes in meditation before breakfast. It's perhaps the most difficult thing I have ever tried to do. In principle it is so simple. I just sit in a good meditation position, and then try to focus my attention only on my breathing. Doesn't sound very difficult, does it? My mind wanders off certainly ten times in ten minutes. What I really should do to get proficient is simply spend more time at it. But the combination of laziness and the dispirited feeling after ten minutes of struggling send me off for a cup of coffee, and then it is on to the order of the day.

My wife is a yoga teacher; she is fortunate to come from a school where the value of the physical exercises, whilst recognised, is subsidiary to the real goal of yoga, which is meditation until one reaches a state of enlightenment. Last year she went to the Himalayas with her school to study with her teacher's guru. There they had a very strict regime and no internet or Facebook to distract them. The time she spent meditating there, the absence of distractions and perhaps the presence of a highly developed spiritual person, gave her the chance to experience what meditation could bring. This was a sort of spring-plank to help her continue the practice at home, and a very valuable, perhaps life-changing experience. She has never, before or since, experienced the peace she felt there.

As I was muddling along with my ten minutes of frustration, I looked for alternative ways which might fit my temperament of being a doer, and not being easily able to sit without having something to do. I came to Tai Chi. This is a combination of meditation whilst being physically active. It gives me my moments of quiet meditation on the movements I am making, and as a bonus is good for maintaining strength and a sense of balance — both useful as one gets older. Even more important, it fits more easily with my nature than pure meditation does, and I enjoy it. One should not underestimate the importance of finding a way to peace of mind which is enjoyable. For me it has meant the difference between struggling and often failing to find the discipline, and now doing my Tai Chi every day without fail, and with enjoyment.

Take-home message

We should do well to realise that our brains, like our bodies, have a finite amount of energy, and to look to focus that energy where we most need it. Mindfulness, meditation yoga, Tai-chi, and gardening are some of the most valuable ways we can spend our time — for mental and physical health. Choosing an activity which gives you enjoyment is the best way to ensure that you will keep it up.

A professor held up an empty pot to his students and filled it with pebbles. "Is it full?" he asked. Most thought it was. He then poured sand into the pot which filled up the spaces between the pebbles. "Is it now full?" he asked. The students were getting careful, but most thought it was now full. The professor poured a cup of coffee into the pot.

The lesson is that if we first fill up our lives with the grains of sand that are Facebook, e-mail and so on, then there will be no time or energy for the important things in life.

Terminal Mushrooms

One recent development in patient care fascinates me. After many years of being frowned upon, psychedelic drugs are being seriously investigated for the treatment of anxiety and depression in terminal cancer patients. In the fifties and sixties of the last century, there was a lot of investigation into LSD and other drugs. Misuse and bad trips led to such drugs being banned, and this was probably a case of throwing the baby away with the bathwater.

Recent studies are showing that, when given to carefully screened terminal cancer patients in a tailored, supportive setting, a single dose of the mushroom extract psilocybin and the subsequent psychedelic experience can lead to enormous improvements in the quality of life. Patients usually experienced something so like the descriptions of mystical experience, including a feeling of 'oneness' with everything and universal love, that it can hardly be coincidence. This experience is apparently so 'mind-blowing' that some sort of mental 'reset' seems to happen. Patients are able to view their situation from a greater emotional distance, and in the majority of cases the fear of death and the associated depression seem to dissolve. Some patients in the trials said that after the treatment they had an unparalleled period of happiness, despite their situation.

One can have long discussions about whether the psychedelic experience has any thing to do with 'truth,' but personally I think such discussions are a waste of time. The only people who may have some claim to know what is and is not true are the advanced yogis, who are reputed to have direct access to knowledge. Although I have my doubts about this, it has to be said that the eastern mystical traditions have made some pretty prescient observations over a period of more than a thousand years, including on the nature of matter. For mere mortals, the truth in this sense will never be knowable. So we have to do with the pragmatic facts: true experience or not, if it is possible to give terminal patients a significant boost in the quality of life for their remaining time, then I'm all for it.

Of great interest to me is the discovery of an area of the brain, called the 'default-mode network' which connects parts of the cortex with much older brain structures like the limbic system. This area seems to be responsible for the feelings of 'self' or ego. fMRI studies have shown that the activity in this brain area is damped down by psilocybin, which fits in very neatly with the experience that the self dissolves and becomes part of the universal whole. What people then experience is apparently identical with descriptions given by mystics and yogis, although the experience often transcends what can be put into words.

It is no surprise then that fMRI studies of people in deep meditation show the same damping down of the default mode network. I hardly dare put this into writing, but my best guess would be that mystics and yogis have found that by many years of discipline and meditation, they can change their brain function in a way that suppresses the sense of self, and gives these experiences of bliss. And it seems likely that you can achieve the same life-changing experience with a single dose of psilocybin! I have always felt that the 'quick-fix' route was rather like getting to the top of a mountain with a helicopter instead of climbing it, and that the discipline and hard work of climbing was just as important as reaching the peak. No place for drugs, I thought, puritanically. But now I wonder. What is coming out of new, well performed research makes me think more along the lines of "get the life changing experience, and then get on and enjoy life, instead of spending it in a cold cave up in the Himalayas!"

I accept that I may well be missing something here. It is clear to me that drugs like psilocybin should only be used under exceptionally well-controlled circumstances. Bad trips seem to occur often when the subject is confronted with a traumatic experience that had been hidden for years. Confronting this 'monster' is paired with fear, which may be extreme, and needs expert guidance. However, when once confronted, the monster may

135

be gone for good. (This is probably similar to the "bad trips" some experience with mindful meditation, as I mentioned earlier.)

Investigations are also under way with treatment of depression and addiction, and preliminary results are promising. In depression the drug seems to cause a resetting of the mind, just as we have to do with a computer which has got stuck. I wonder if that is why electro-convulsive therapy works? For people wanting to stop smoking, it looks as if treatment with psilocybin may give a far higher success rate than conventional therapy.

It's early days yet, and of course there are concerns with misuse and control of such drugs. This damping down of the ego might be worthwhile in itself for some of the colleagues I am writing about, but whether you want them treating patients whilst high on psilocybin is another matter!

What I seriously would love to see is a study of 100 "problem" specialists in which half are given a single treatment with psilocybin under supportive care, and then document the behaviour of both groups over a six month period. Such a study will probably never be carried out, but if did happen, then I anticipate very interesting and telling results

Take home message

This much is clear to me: if ever I suffer anxiety and depression with terminal cancer, then bring on the mushrooms!

"Stephen kissed me in the spring,
Robin in the fall,
But Colin only looked at me
And never kissed at all.

Stephen's kiss was lost in jest,
Robin's lost in play,
But the kiss in Colin's eyes
Haunts me night and day"

Sara Teasdale, The Collected Poems

The body can heal itself

Homeopathy

We doctors tend to have the idea, and to propagate it, that people who are ill need a doctor to get better, and unfortunately many patients agree with this. We doctors do have a place, but it is also true that the body has its own healing mechanisms, and we often tend to forget that. Like many things in life, our health shows upward and downward swings. Our immune system shows the same pattern. When we get the flu, we expect to get sick, and also to get better again, and most people realise that we will get better again with or without a doctor. Our moods tend to swing up and down, and usually settle back to our average state. Our abilities show this same pattern: our performance swings up and down over a given period, and with no intervention tends to return to our average performance.

In his brilliant book "Thinking fast and slow," Kahneman describes this phenomenon. It is called regression toward the mean and has led to some interesting misunderstandings. For instance some teachers noticed that when they gave their students praise, their performance tended to be worse the next time, and when they were highly critical, then performance improved. This fits entirely with the expectations that our results tend to swing around the average. However the teachers drew the conclusion that their praise led to reduced performance, and criticism to improvement. For them it was clear; you can better be critical of your students than praise them. I cannot think of a clearer example of how we can draw conclusions from what we observe that may be completely wrong.

Probably this mechanism also explains why people believe so emphatically in homeopathy; they have some small health problem, and they get better again. If they have taken some potion (even if it is just water with a "memory" of some magic substance), they will credit it with having cured them. Perhaps strangely, if they take the potion and get worse, this does not usually lead to any less belief in its effectiveness. Our minds work in wondrous ways!

To laugh often and much;
to win the respect of intelligent people
and the affection of children;
to earn the appreciation of honest
critics and endure the betrayal of false
friends;
to appreciate beauty;
to find the best in others;
to leave the world a bit better, whether
by a healthy child, a garden patch or a
redeemed social condition;
to know even one life has breathed
easier because you have lived.
That is to have succeeded.

Emerson

Afraid to learn

Most humans have capacities which remain largely undeveloped. Many other animals are born with the software already installed; a foal does not need to learn to walk, or make the sounds it will use. These are pre-programmed, as it were. Ninety-nine percent of horses will not develop their motor skills beyond what they need: walking, trotting and galloping. There remains untapped potential for motor development; think of dressage, for instance, but it is relatively limited.

The human, in contrast, is born free of much of this "software," which is developed through the process of learning. A baby is born without a language module. This makes for a slow start, but leaves the baby free to write its own software, as it were, for the particular language it needs. Usually, once we have learned our own language sufficiently to express our needs, we stop learning, and the growth curve levels out. In so doing, we leave an enormous potential untapped. We have the capacity to learn many languages. Cardinal Giuseppe Caspar Mezzofanti, born in 1774, spoke 38 languages and 40 dialects. Similarly, we learn to walk and run, and many leave it at that. Many of us add motor skills like playing an instrument, or playing a sport, but again, the potential for growth is phenomenal: think of a performer from Cirque Du Soleil, or a Swiss watchmaker assembling a complicated timepiece. We can only conclude that we have an enormous reservoir of potential in our brains and bodies.

It is such a pity then that we so often limit ourselves by thinking, "I cannot draw," or, "I'm hopeless at mathematics". One story sticks in my mind about two teenage boys who have skipped the maths class because they are no good at it. They are outside throwing a ball to each other. Just consider the maths involved in calculating the force and trajectory necessary to do that! The ability is there but untapped by the conscious mind. There are individual limits; recent work suggests that our genes account for about 70% of our potential for academic growth, and that the choice of school, and all the changes and fads in the teaching world only account for about twenty percent of the difference between children. However, within these inborn limits, most people still have tremendous room for growth which is never developed.

One limitation for growth is our environment. A child might have great potential for playing a musical instrument; imagine the different outcomes if he or she is born into a family with a piano and musical traditions, or one without either the instrument or the interest.

Another important environmental factor can be statements made by key people during our early development. A teacher who says, "You will never learn to draw" probably does not realise that he has just implanted a belief in the young brain. And if you believe that you cannot draw, why should you take the trouble? It is only once someone makes us conscious that this is largely self-limitation that we have a chance to reconsider our beliefs, and discover just how well we can draw after all.

There is another factor which limits learning and growth; I saw it at work yesterday, and that is the vulnerable ego. We had a patient with very difficult veins. Three of us had tried and failed to set up an intravenous infusion. One of the anaesthetic assistants told us that one of his colleagues had worked in a specialised team in a university hospital, just for such cases. He had a great deal of experience using ultrasound. He was present in the theatre complex, and we got him to help us. Using ultrasound, he got the infusion running at the first attempt.

And now here's the point; he had offered to teach the technique to his colleagues, but this offer had been turned down because some of the anaesthetists were against it. This is where ego gets in the way of learning. Someone like this assistant is a valuable asset to an anaesthetic department; such a pity that he is seen as a threat to the ego of some specialists. My approach would be, "Teach it to anyone who wants to learn, but teach me first!" I am certain that insecurity lies at the roots of this story, and I have seen it so often. In this case there is the added complication that the assistant in question seems to take himself very seriously, and wants others to know that he is a cut above the rest, and this does tend to alienate people, and make it harder for them to learn from him. Just why we don't like people who show off is an interesting story in itself, but it should not get in the way of learning.

Many of us have our little areas of expertise; someone with no ego problem will seek such people out and learn from them, and in so doing become a better and more all-round doctor, and incidentally also a happier doctor, because growth feeds happiness. My own area of expertise is regional anaesthesia. I have a great deal of experience, and I know that my nerve blocks are better than most. I am present as a locum in a department for a limited time. A few of the junior colleagues have used this opportunity to learn the "tips and tricks" I can give them. The result is that their nerve blocks are better than those of most of the colleagues who have not done so. (To keep it in perspective, I am also well aware that outside my "niche" area, you would sometimes be better off with one of my colleagues than with me.) What saddens me a bit is to see that many colleagues have shown no interest whatsoever in trying to find out what it is that I do differently that leads to better results, and thus safer and happier patients. At the end of a six months period I was gone, taking my little packet of expertise with me, plus all the new things I have learned. Unfortunately most of my colleagues will have learned nothing from my presence, and will continue to have many more failed nerve blocks than is necessary. Is it disinterest, or ego, or lack of awareness about their own success rate? I don't know. Or is it just my own ego inflating my own value?

One reason why I still enjoy my work at the age of 70 is that I still love learning, and am prepared to learn from the cleaning lady if she can teach me something useful, even if it's only that it's handier to put the cup-a-soup powder in first and then add the hot water instead of the other way around.

Take-home message

One key to fulfilment in life is to retain the inquisitive attitude of those learning machines called children. Once we have learned enough to get by, many of us stop asking questions, and to some extent stop growing. And when growth stops, disintegration starts and we never achieve our full potential.

Courage is doing what you are afraid
to do. There can be no courage unless
you're scared

Eddie Rickenbacker

Cognitive dissonance

The downfall of a university department.

C ognitive dissonance is a very uncomfortable feeling, which we will go to great lengths to avoid. And just how far we are prepared to go to avoid that feeling has amazed me.

Cognitive dissonance occurs when we try to keep two mutually incompatible ideas in our head at the same time. For instance I might think of myself as a caring and competent doctor. I may also have unwittingly caused the deaths of patients. Knowledge of these two things would cause negative tension, and this is cognitive dissonance. If someone were to point out to me how many deaths I had caused, how far would I be prepared to go to reduce that uncomfortable feeling? Would I be prepared to let more patients die? What a preposterous suggestion! Unfortunately, preposterous or not, it has happened, and will continue to happen.

In the mid 18th century many women died from puerperal fever (an infection following on childbirth). An interesting observation was that the chance of dying was far higher if the delivery was carried out by a doctor than when it was carried out by a midwife. The distinguished Dr. Semmelweis wondered how this could be. Although at that time bacteria and viruses had yet to be discovered, he made the connection between doctors carrying out autopsies on the women who had just died and then returning directly to the delivery room to deliver the next baby. He instructed his assistants to wash their hands before attending to the next patient, and the death rate dropped dramatically. One would expect that his findings would have made a deep impression, and that his colleagues would have thanked him, and followed his example. In practice, they ignored his findings, and simply said that he was wrong. This seems to be quite inexplicable, but the theory of cognitive dissonance tells us that they were unable to cope with rhyming the fact that they were directly responsible for the unnecessary deaths of many women with their belief in themselves as caring and competent doctors. Semmelweis died in a psychiatric institution at the age of 47. It was many years after his death before his insight was applied in medicine. A clearer example of the doctor's ego leading to the death of patients is hard to imagine.

A very logical approach would have been if his colleagues had said to themselves "even though I am a good and caring doctor, I am not infallible and I have learnt something new which will help me to save hundreds of lives." However the sad fact is that for the great majority, this simple idea of being fallible is intolerable. The only other way to reduce the feeling of dissonance was to convince themselves that the findings were simply wrong. And it is amazing how creative we can be when we try to convince ourselves that something bent is straight, or vice versa. And so patients continued to die in order to prevent the doctors from feeling too uncomfortable. The idea that being wrong is equivalent to being stupid, and that it is thus associated with identity, apparently varies from culture to culture. In some cultures, being wrong is just a part of the process of learning, and one would anticipate that cognitive dissonance would play a smaller part in such societies.

Well, fortunately, we have advanced a lot since the 1850s. Or have we? I am writing at a time when something quite comparable seems to be happening in one of our university hospitals. There follows an account which is a mixture of the facts as I understand them with my interpretations of those facts in the light of cognitive dissonance and self-justification. My purpose here is not to write history, but to demonstrate the underlying psychological mechanisms.

For a perfect example of cognitive dissonance, I recommend studying how the Republican party and senators are behaving in the impeachment proceedings against Donald Trump.

How power, cognitive dissonance, and self-justification can lead to the ruin of a good department

The ENT Department of an academic teaching hospital ran along happily with a highly respected head of department with a good track record, including important developments in cochlea implantation. A new professor was placed at the head of the department, and got the support of the hospital management as he promised improvements in efficiency and income from the department. The previous head of department was careful in selecting patients for cochlear implantation. The new head of department increased the number of patients by widening the selection criteria. He also introduced short-cuts in the technique so that the operations could be carried out quicker. (this has had disastrous effects on some patients). This policy was opposed by the previous head of department who lost his position as a result. The new professor not only increased the number of implantation patients, but also insisted on a higher work tempo, which some of his staff members considered to be dangerous. Over the course of the next few years two patients died unexpectedly during or shortly after operations, one because the carotid artery was accidentally cut, and the other because of an uncontrollable bleeding in the nose. Neither of these calamities was reported to the Health Inspectors despite the fact that failing to do so in the Netherlands is a criminal act punishable with three years imprisonment. In one case the patient's dossier described the death as due to natural causes. In law this declaration may only be given after post-mortem examination by a medical examiner. Investigative journalists from a television programme later discovered that no such doctor had ever examined the patient in question.

A young doctor, a new member of the ENT staff, was concerned about this, and the fact that there was an atmosphere of fear in the department, and a pressure to carry out operations at an irresponsible tempo. He, and one or two other doctors expressed their concerns in repeated contacts

148

with the hospital's confidential counsellor. The hospital management later denied any knowledge of these contacts. The doctors approached the hospital inspectors in connection with the situation in the department and the two calamities. Out of fear of retribution they refused to name the patients, and the management falsely reassured the inspectors that there had been no incidents which should have been reported. Other doctors in the department told the inspectors that the head of department set high standards, but that there were no problems. The inspector dropped the matter. The hospital management then reported the whistle-blower to the inspectors! They found no grounds to the hospital's complaints, and issued no sanctions against the doctor concerned. Following on this, the professor declared that they would examine which doctors brought in the most money for the department, and surprise, surprise, the young doctor was found not to be productive enough, and was fired. He later found work in the UK, where he works to general satisfaction. Members of the medical staff interviewed by the inspectors claimed that there was no question of intimidation or dangerous practices in the department.

Are you starting to shake your head in disbelief? Eventually the story was leaked to investigative journalists, who confronted the hospital's director for quality and safety. Never have I seen a man so lost for words as he was in the interview. It gave the strong impression that he knew what was going on, and was obliged to tell the world that everything was just fine. There were also damming interviews with the dismissed doctor, and the professor who had been "edged out" of the department. The head of the national ENT association gave his judgement that there was no excuse whatsoever for not reporting the deaths to the inspectors, and another professor in quality and safety spoke of "falsification of documents". The ENT association and the inspectors announced new investigations.

My first thought was that the hospital management would now have to come clean, and get things sorted out. In the first place it would seem inevitable that many patients would cancel their operations in a department where such things were going on. At any rate, there was sufficient reason to be concerned that unnecessary operations might be being carried out. More importantly, additional loss of life might occur if the departmental procedures continued unchanged. To my initial surprise the management only counter-attacked by saying that they would be taking legal proceedings against those who had leaked the information, that there were no new facts in the TV programme, and that they saw no reason to doubt the safety and efficiency of the department. In other words, complete denial.

Immediately before the television programme was aired, the hospital decided perhaps it might be a good idea to report the two unexpected deaths to the Inspectorate (nothing to do with the upcoming TV programme, of course). On the same day that the programme was aired, twenty-four out of the twenty-five doctors in the department signed a joint letter stating that they did not recognise themselves in the television programme's findings, and that there was no reason to question patient safety in the examples given. Given the facts, this was a fairly astounding declaration, and can only be attributed to dishonesty or cognitive dissonance.

As this news broke, I was reading a book on cognitive dissonance titled "Mistakes were made, (but not by me)" by Carol Tavris and Elliot Aronson, and all at once everything fell into place. I can imagine that it might go like this (and it might not have gone like this at all; this is after all, my imagination!) The management names a new head of department, who is going to be a new broom and clean out the department, improve its efficiency and increase its earnings. Management gets behind the professor for these highly desirable changes. The professor starts to deliver; by modifying the selection procedure for a lucrative implant operation, the department starts to bring in more money and by pressuring medical staff to operate more quickly, the production from the department is increased. Management sees that they have done the right thing by backing this head of department, even if it has led to the loss of one of their prominent surgeons because he felt unable to go along with the new selection procedures and operating pressures. Having convinced themselves that they were right to back him, management starts to look only for evidence which supports their decision, and fails to register complaints coming from within the department that all is not well. Gradually the head of department becomes more and more tyrannical but management ignores signals about this. When a young member of staff blows the whistle, management turns on him; after all, they were right in standing behind their professor, and so any negative signals must be wrong. This doctor, with his negative stories, is damaging the department. They hit back against the young man by informing the inspectorate that he is the problem, and even though the inspector finds nothing against him, the head of department hits on a plan to get rid of him: he refuses to comply with what he considers as dangerous work-practices, with the result that he works more slowly than demanded. This means that he is bringing in less money for the department, and this is used as an excuse to get rid of him. To any right minded person this is crazy policy, but once you have gone so far down the road of self justification it seems quite sensible. Otherwise you might just have to admit that you had been wrong.

Cognitive dissonance theory also explains why the large majority of doctors in the department signed the letter denying that there were any problems with quality. When the Inspectorate carried out an investigation after the whistleblowing episode, the other doctors claimed to a man that there was nothing wrong. This is not entirely surprising if indeed the department was subject to a regime of intimidation, and certainly not after having seen one of their colleagues who had the courage to stand up for his convictions kicked out. On the occasion of the television broadcast, it is entirely possible that the same motivation kept the doctors quiet. Cognitive dissonance would account for the fact that having told the inspectors that nothing was wrong, it was now extremely difficult to turn round three years later and admit that you had been lying to save your own skin. So the specialists in the Department probably convinced themselves that there wasn't really anything seriously wrong.

In these matters there comes a breaking point. After the phase of indignation and self-righteousness, the pressure from outside builds. Awkward questions start being asked from all sides: inspectors, E.N.T. society, patient groups and of course increasing internal rumblings and rumours. The facade starts to crack. It never breaks open with a declaration: "we have been wrong, and should have taken action long ago," just small awkward steps to make sure that the ice doesn't break underfoot. "We have decided to appoint an external commission to investigate the situation as a result of internal signals" (in other words, not as a result of the television programme's

151

revelations). A week later we learn that the head of department and the surgeon responsible for the two deaths have been "given leave of absence". Months later the head of department decides to "stand down." "Gentle doctors make stinking wounds" is an apt comparison to the way the management approached the situation. This has all the appearances of another clear example of the individual ego of a head of department leading to the death of patients, and also the complicity of the collective ego of the medical staff and the hospital management.

Without taking account of self-justification, the actions of management and the department seem completely inexplicable; however in the light of cognitive dissonance, their behaviour is entirely logical. In the long term, of course, it is not the most appropriate or sensible way of behaving. Far better would have been to admit that they, management and head of department, had made very serious mistakes, and that they would now be taking action to correct this.   Going, as they did, into denial gave them some respite in the short term, but guaranteed that further down the road, more medical mishaps would occur, with possibly very severe financial consequences. Assuming the correctness of my interpretations, this would certainly not be the first case in which hospital management ignored blatantly obvious problems until eventually the ship sunk with them still at the helm. Outsiders were left shaking their heads and wondering how it was possible that it could have gone so far. With knowledge of cognitive dissonance and self-justification, it is no longer a surprise — just a disappointment.

As far as I am aware, no legal measures were taken against the management, despite the fact that the law had been broken.

I can imagine that cognitive dissonance and self-justification are the most important reasons why whistleblowers are almost universally treated so badly by their employers. In their state of self denial, the employers can only see the whistleblowers as troublemakers determined to ruin the organisation. At the same time, these people are seen by outsiders to be the rare examples of employees with the courage to stand up for what they believe in. They often end up in poverty and without work, which seems desperately unfair. That's why I'm glad that in this case the whistleblower was able to establish a new future, albeit in another country.

As mentioned earlier, "Power tends to corrupt, and absolute power corrupts absolutely." We usually think of it in political terms, but it applies to every situation in which one person has power over others. The word "tends" is here of importance; it points out that corruption through power is not inevitable. However, in the long term, there is a strong tendency for a leader to increasingly surround himself with people who support his own opinions and beliefs (it is usually a man). There have been a few rare cases in history when leaders deliberately added people to their close circle who *disagreed* with them: Abraham Lincoln was apparently one such example. It demands courage and strength of character to do this, and unfortunately most leaders gradually eliminate such tiresome people from their immediate circle. This inevitably gives them a highly skewed view of reality and explains the many African leaders who once were against life presidents until they took over that position themselves and gradually became convinced that it was after all for the good of the country. They then did everything they could, including changing the Constitution, to stay in power. Their track record would seem to suggest that this is perhaps not such a good idea after all. As I write, there is a president in America who, I suspect, would love to become an autocrat, on the lines of Putin of Russia and Erdogan or Turkey, and he is actually making quite good progress in this direction (August 2018).

I would suggest that cognitive dissonance is probably the cause of about 80% of communication problems, inside and outside the hospital setting with poor communication techniques coming a close second. Humanity is capable of some really stupid actions that are often institutionalised and highly damaging. And we are even more expert in creating stories to explain why these actions are really entirely sensible. Let me just give three examples of this.

The Dinka tribe in southern Sudan extract the front teeth of their children as part of a coming-of-age ritual. This unpleasant habit is usually carried out without anaesthetic, and causes cosmetic and speech changes. Most

153

members of the tribe are quite unaware of the origins of this habit. It probably started in the time that tetanus, otherwise known as lockjaw, was a frequently occurring infection. It could be impossible to feed someone with lockjaw, and the solution they found for this was to remove the front teeth. Although this origin is unknown to most of the people who undergo the procedure, they will yet come with a number of arguments which they find persuasive as to why the habit should be continued. They may support it with arguments about adulthood, beauty, tribal identity, sound production, and soft food consumption. One could consider tribal identity as being the one possibly sensible argument in that series.

For a period of some 700 years it was the habit to bind the feet of upper-class Chinese women. There are various explanations for the origins of this barbaric habit which left women in constant pain and almost unable to walk. Part of the procedure was to fold the toes underneath the foot, and put so much pressure on to them that the toes would break. About 600 years ago a Chinese intellectual remarked that he found it hard to find any sense in this ritual, but it took until 1912 before it was banned. Foot binding became so institutionalised that it was pretty well unthinkable for a high-class woman to find a husband if her feet had not been bound. There were a number of justifications for this procedure, among them the claim that it was erotic. However the husbands did not often actually want to see the bound feet, or to smell them, as it was more or less impossible to wash them effectively! But the idea was considered to be erotic.

Female genital mutilation is perhaps the most horrific example in this row of completely useless and cruel rituals. Although being banned officially in most countries, it is still carried out on a large-scale causing untold suffering and even death. Again many arguments will be proffered to demonstrate that this is really in the best interests of the girls involved.

Each of these examples must involve a considerable degree of cognitive dissonance. Imagine trying to keep in your head at the same time the idea that you are a caring and loving mother and yet you let someone cut off your daughter's clitoris with an unsterile razor blade and then stitch the perineum together in such a way that only urinating is possible. I think that if I

154

was that mother, it would cause a fair degree of cognitive dissonance which would force me to find some compelling arguments, in which I could believe implicitly, for why I am allowing this to happen.

The above examples have a number of things in common. To start with they are all, seen objectively, completely useless, harmful, painful and in some cases deadly. Seen through the eyes of an objective observer, these habits are completely inexplicable, and yet they will all be explained and defended with a religious fervour. Because of the cognitive dissonance, the person involved doesn't just try to convince the outside world of the rightness of what they are doing, but far more importantly they convince *themselves*. Communication between the outsider and the insider is then pretty well impossible and this explains why it can take hundreds of years to change such rituals.

These are shocking examples, and serve to illustrate clearly what is going on. However it is of great importance to realise that cognitive dissonance plays a part in all of us albeit in a less horrific way. We all make mistakes and do bad things from time to time, and our natural reaction is to defend what we do and find explanations to lower the internal tension they cause.

One example of this is when a teenage girl gets put under peer pressure to bully another girl. On the way home she will probably experience cognitive dissonance; I am a really nice girl and I did a really nasty thing. The natural response is regrettably that she will convince herself that the bullied girl deserved this in some way. This reduces the internal tension and incidentally makes it easier for the bullying to escalate the next day. If the parent tries to talk with the daughter about this, then it will probably be a difficult conversation as the daughter has already convinced herself that she was in the right.

The above is just an illustration. The important thing to realise is that this is something we all do to a greater or lesser extent. The less self-worth we have, I suspect the more we shall demonstrate this behaviour.

It is so hard to do the only sensible thing, which will relieve the internal tension and allow us to put it behind us, and that is to say, "I did a bad thing, I'm sorry"

There have been occasions when this latter approach has been tried, and with great success. I suppose the best example is the truth and reconciliation council after the apartheid era in South Africa.

Take-home message

Knowledge about cognitive dissonance is important for two reasons. It helps us to explain the behaviour of others, and it helps us to recognise this process in ourselves, and hopefully to change it.

I like long walks, especially when they
are taken by people who annoy me.

Fred Alan

On call

B eing on call for the hospital has been part of my life from my first hospital job until my sixtieth year. Among the many changes I have encountered in my time, probably nothing has changed more drastically than finding the doctor in the first place.

Before the invention of the telephone, finding your GP could be a daunting task. Probably best to saddle up the horse and gallop round to his house. "He's up at Dawson's farm, and after that he was going to have a look at grandma Griffith up on the heath". By the time you get to grandma, she is able to tell you that the doctor was called down to Mrs Smith who was having one of her turns. One wonders how many lives were lost before the doctor was eventually found in bed with young Betty Carson - "just to comfort her, what with her Fred going off with her best friend"

When I started, we at least had the telephone, but being on call largely meant staying at home or in the hospital. A visit to a friend close by was possible as long as you gave the telephone number to the receptionist. It wasn't foolproof; I remember that when I was on duty for two hospitals in Winterswijk in the Netherlands, the police were battering on the door of my house in the middle of the night. I was giving an anaesthetic for a caesarian section in one hospital, but the other hospital didn't think to look for me there when I did not answer at home. Some may say that I should have informed them of my whereabouts, but cognitive dissonance prevents me from admitting that. When on duty, one did not go shopping, or for a walk, and I was on duty every other night, and every other weekend.

What a relief it was when technology came to my assistance in the form of a semaphone. This was an object the size of a book with an extendable antenna. This thing was incredibly advanced: it had three lights, one to show that the reception was o.k., one to say that I had to go to the hospital at

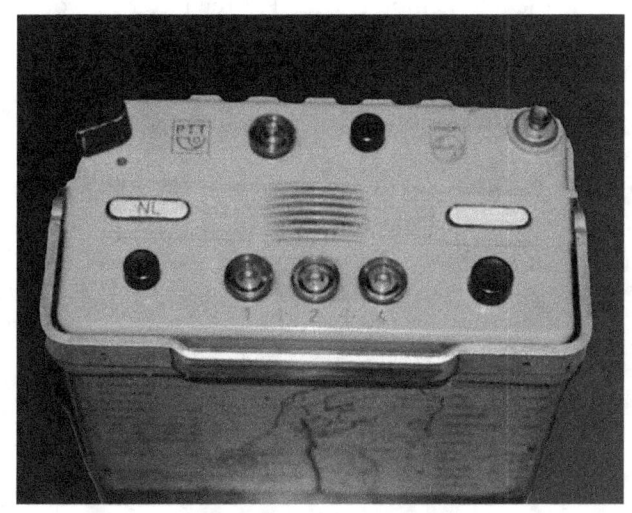

once, and one to say that I should ring the hospital. The light showing reception was essential. Although I was now free to go to the bakery on a Saturday morning, I had to hang around near the window, as I would

Old model semaphone

otherwise lose reception. This was no small matter: if I was unavailable, it could literally cost a life, as there was often no other anaesthetist in town and there was no other way of finding me, so the feeling of freedom was limited by the fact that I was constantly looking to see if that little light was

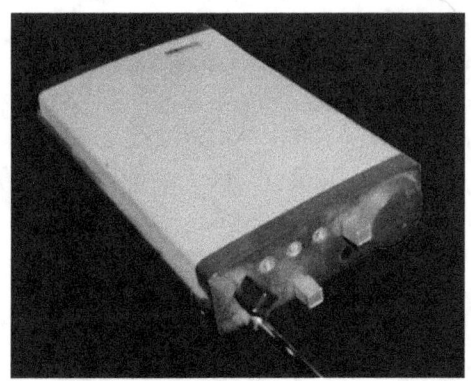

giving me the o.k. On the other hand, this large object did give me a certain status, and I probably had to wait less long for my croissants than the average person. I can still see that large cheery baker's wife telling a German doctor's wife from just across the border that she would have to wait until I had been served. This did not go down

Intermediate model

well; a doctor's wife in Germany at that time expected to be addressed as, "frau dokter," and to be treated with deference. A lot of people in Winterswijk still had bitter memories of the war, and many of them, like this bak-

159

er's wife, did not try to hide their contempt. Having left the bakery, I would move on to the next shop, only to discover that I had left the semaphone in the window of the bakery where it at least had reception. Then I would run back with some feeling of panic, in case I had missed a vital call.

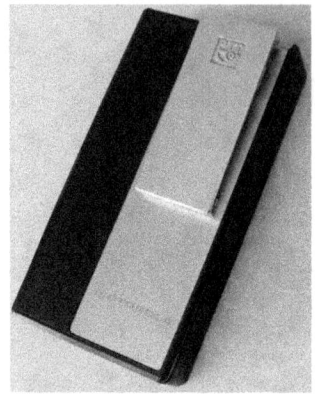

later model semaphone

I digress; as the years went by the semaphone shrunk, as did my associated status. In the end it was the size of my thumb, and I was treated as if I was an ordinary human being. (Fortunately this let down was gradual; when I started as a junior doctor in 1972, a dear little nun would bring me coffee and cake on a silver tray; now I walk 100 meters to the coffee room, and a machine pours my coffee into a plastic cup — and, as you willunderstand, no silver tray to carry it back on.)

But the semaphone had still not learned to tell me more than that I should ring or run.

Then the big breakthrough came: the mobile phone. Well, I say mobile, but that may give the wrong impression. It was the size of a small aircraft cabin case, and very heavy. In our town only the hospital physician possessed such a high tech and expensive piece of apparatus. When Christmas approached a small select group was invited to cut down their own Christmas tree in the wood owned by one of the surgeons. It took a while before I achieved this elevated status, but I shall never forget my first mobile phone call, and it was in this wood. The physician lugged her phone with her (so that someone else had to carry her tree). She called me over, and it was the on-duty surgeon who wanted to remove an appendix; would I mind going to the hospital. Well I did mind, but I went.

Fast forward to today, when I can be reached almost anywhere in the world, read books, check the internet, navigate, do my banking, take photographs and a hundred and one other things with the mobile phone I can fit in my pocket.

Well, It's certainly progress, and it's certainly not conducive to mindfulness!

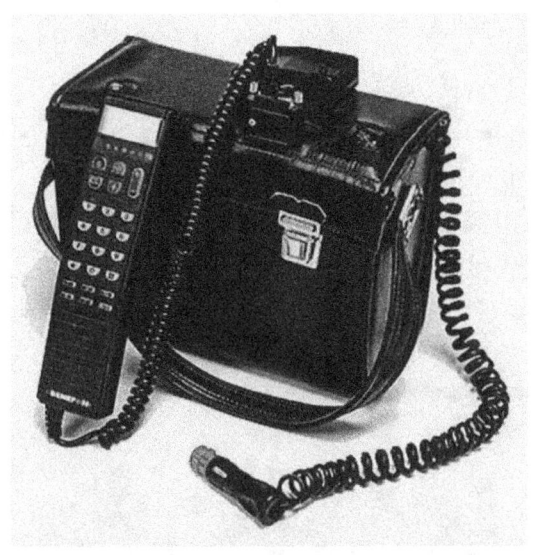

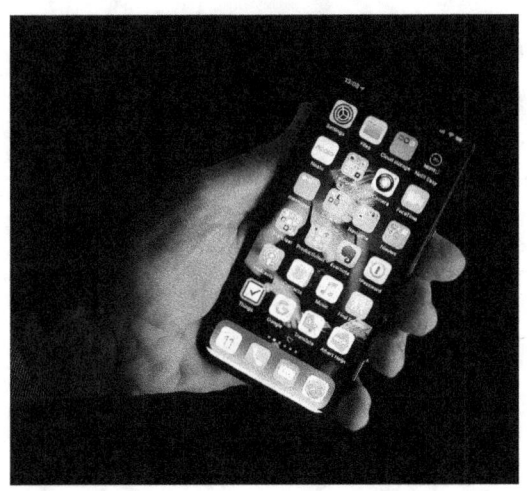

> Basically my wife was immature. I'd be at home in the bath and she'd come in and sink my boats.

Woody Allan

Medical Missers

One of the most important changes in my time as a doctor is the disappearance of the small cottage hospitals, and perhaps more importantly the disappearance of the solo-working medical specialist. This was generally a good development. I have seen some things to make the blood run cold, and sometimes it did.

In the town where I lived and worked for twenty-four years, we had two surgeons, and they were fine. I should not have liked a broken leg to be operated on by one of them, but in general they were competent and conscientious. I was on duty one weekend and a young man, the son of a local policeman, was brought in after a car accident. On admission he was in a stable condition, and we called in the surgeon from the next small hospital, who was covering for the weekend. He asked some questions, and decided that it would not be necessary to come. A hour later it was clear that something major was going on, and I called the surgeon again. He refused to come and examine the patient himself. I felt that there was internal bleeding going on, and decided to stick a needle into the abdomen. I aspirated pure blood, and called the surgeon again. With this information the surgeon decided that he <u>definitely</u> wanted nothing to do with this patient. "He will probably die on the table, and I don't want that." There was no one else at hand to call, apart from the hospital director. I considered putting the patient in an ambulance to the nearest large hospital, but estimated that he would not survive the trip. This would almost certainly have been the case as the young man died needlessly shortly after my last call. Another case of the Doctor's ego leading to a death which might well have been prevented. We made a complaint to the directorate, and I never saw the surgeon again, but heard that he was at work somewhere in Germany, leaving something of a tax debt and a case for medical negligence behind him. Although I have fortunately never been confronted with this degree of negligence again, I have seen plenty of incompetence.

The worst case of incompetence I experienced wasn't negligence, but it *was* fatal. I was giving anaesthesia for a caesarian section which delivered premature twins. One of these was in a bad way and I called our paediatrician in. In the meantime I put a tube into the airway of one child in order to assist respiration. The paediatrician was a man of about sixty years; pretty experienced, you may think. He asked me to have the babies taken up to the children's ward. When the section was finished I went to see how the babies were doing. The one I had intubated was dead. I asked what had happened. The paediatrician had connected the tube directly to the oxygen outlet, with no reservoir bag or valve in between. This was unforgivable and amazingly incompetent. A first year's medical student would have realised that this would have caused the lungs to explode in an instant. This doctor was put out to grass shortly after.

Next in line was our orthopaedic surgeon. He had many years experience, was loved by his patients, and was a pretty hopeless operator. Patients would hobble into his outpatient clinic after he had muddled through another hip replacement. He would ask how they were getting on, and that was often not very well. His explanation was that their hip was so badly damaged that it was a miracle that they could walk at all! And off they went, so relieved that they had found such a brilliant surgeon. At one point he put a prosthetic bone back to front in a wrist, taking no notice of the warning of the assisting nurse. After that steps were taken to persuade him to take a well-earned premature retirement. When I say well-earned, I mean that he was probably offered a golden handshake if he would just go quietly. I never knew the details, but he seemed to live quite comfortably.

The final case was our ENT doctor, and I suppose he was about seventy when I worked in the hospital. At that time it was usual for tonsils to be removed by sitting the child on the knees of a nun. The narcotiseur, as the anaesthetist was then called, would push a mask on the unfortunate child's face, and give the anaesthetic gas trichloroethylene. This put the poor

164

struggling creature asleep just long enough for the surgeon to put a spreader in the mouth, and wrench the tonsils out with a guillotine just in time (usually) before the child woke up again, in a state of some displeasure. If the nun's chair was not exactly placed where it should be and at the right angle, then the ENT surgeon became flustered, and could only proceed once conditions had been standardised. He wore a long plastic apron, and under the head mirror on his forehead was a large clear x-ray sheet. He must have looked terrifying to the children.

At one point during an operation on an adult he lost his needle, and I had to find it for him somewhere at the back of the throat. The last straw for me was when he was looking for a foreign body in the throat on another occasion. With a grunt of triumph he said, "I've got it," and he started tugging my endotracheal tube out of the airway. After that he had to be persuaded to limit himself to doing the tonsils, and was thus given a gentle path into retirement.

These cases are in themselves an argument for enlarging the scale of hospitals. Having solo specialists, with their status and power and no one to check on their competence was really a recipe for disaster. These days groups of specialists can monitor each other, and they are regularly visited by a group of peers to see that they are giving the expected quality of care. It is now mandatory for specialists to follow regular post-graduate training courses.

Unfortunately even under these circumstances, peer oversight fails from time to time. One advantage of being on the inside is that I know who to avoid!

Small scale hospitals have the advantage of short lines. Shortly after I started in the Netherlands, an anaesthetist presented his professorial thesis, with the title, "Death on the table". This led to a national committee recommending minimal standards for anaesthetic and monitoring apparatus. I was able to approach the director, and say, "I need this and this and this, and it will cost X thousand guilders." "Okay, go and order it." Those were the days! Now, with all the workgroups, budget holders and commissions there would be a good many more dead on the table before the apparatus arrived.

Take home message

Small hospitals have their advantages — there is more often a family atmosphere, and everyone knows everyone. However the advantages of larger specialist groups with collegial oversight, and sub-specialisation mean that larger scale hospitals will usually deliver a better quality of care.

While there is a chance of the world getting through its troubles, I hold that a reasonable man has to behave as though he were sure of it. If at the end your cheerfulness is not justified, at any rate you will have been cheerful

H. G. Wells

Way out of my depth

What happens when empathy goes too far.

I shall recount the most painful experience of my career. It is an example of how a well meaning doctor can become trapped in a situation in which his emotions are involved, and there seems no way out.

The girl was 18 years old when I first saw her in the pain clinic, some thirty years ago. I shall call her Hester. She came into the room with her parents. She was a very thin girl with a shock of red hair, a pale face and large serous eyes and she walked in on crutches. Father was a somewhat dominant man with glasses and short grey hair, and mother a quiet kindly woman. Hester told me her story with frequent additions from father. Two years earlier she had been kicked in her knee by a horse. At that time she was a passionate show jumper, and full of life.

As a result of the accident she developed a condition known as post-traumatic dystrophy. In this condition, the symptom most in the foreground is severe pain. The affected limb is kept immobile to reduce the pain, and eventually becomes atrophied and stiff. The circulation suffers as well. Neither the cause nor the treatment is well understood. I examined the leg; it was dusky blue, cold and atrophied, with an ulcer on the thigh that would not heal. It was typical of a late stage post-traumatic dystrophy. The diagnosis had been missed by her GP, and he had referred her to a psychiatrist for the "psychic" pain. (This led to Hester having a deep aversion to all psychiatrists and psychologists.) She could walk a little with crutches before the pain became too severe, and cycle with an adapted bicycle.

168

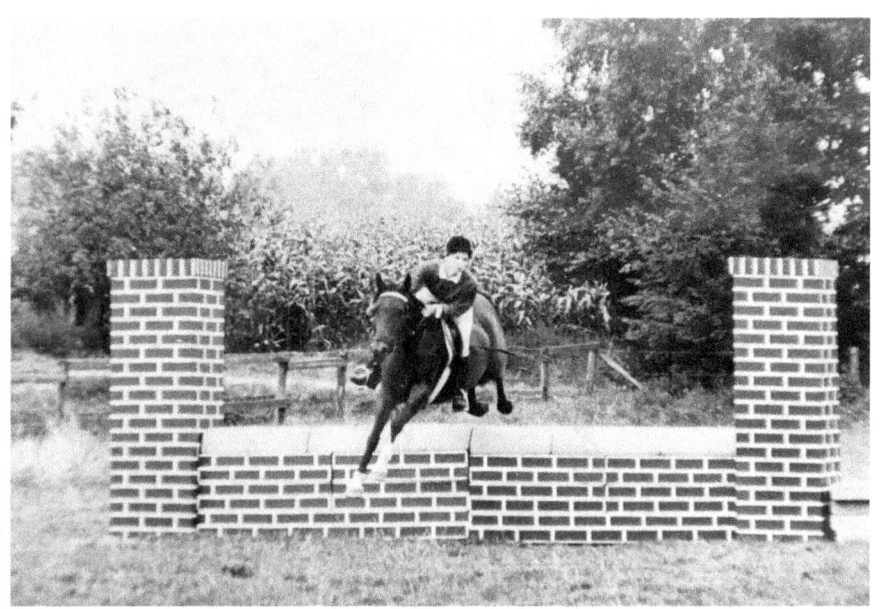

The referring surgeon requested a lumbar sympathetic block to see whether this might alleviate the pain and improve the circulation so that the ulcer might heal. A sympathetic block is a procedure to block the nerves leading to the blood vessels in a limb. It can be a temporary block with a local anaesthetic to test whether it will be effective, or a permanent block if the test helps. I knew that the dystrophy was in a terminal phase, and that it was extremely unlikely to improve with any known therapy.

At that time many treatments were being used with no scientific evidence that they were effective. The most bizarre one was "colour therapy". A number of patients in the Netherlands at that time collected money from friends and family to travel to a "doctor" in New Zealand, who claimed amazing results with dystrophy patients. This man asked them to send a urine sample, which he examined by passing a divining rod over it. This always resulted in the diagnosis of polio! Patients then spent five days and a fair sum of money sitting in a room in his house, with an arm-band connected to a small metal bowl in which there was a coloured silk bundle. The colour of the silk was vital to the success of the therapy, and was also determined using the divining rod. From the other end of the silk, a wire went into a black box. The content of the black box was not made known (that's what black boxes are for!) Some of these patients improved, which to me is a sign of how powerful the placebo effect is. What it does make clear is that we doctors were quite unable to help them, and they had so much pain that they would grasp at any straw. I spoke to the doctor in New Zealand, and he offered to license his system to me for use in the Netherlands. Otherwise he was not able to give me details of his therapy! It could have made me rich, using a treatment carrying no risks, and no on-call duties. Quite a contrast with my daily work as anaesthetist. There was however no way I could have applied this treatment and keep my integrity intact (or my face straight!) but I have to admit that he probably had better results with dystrophy patients than I did. Of course, if you have borrowed a whole lot of money from family and friends for the therapy, you can't really afford not to get better!

I digress. Although it seemed unlikely that a sympathectomy would be of any benefit for the dystrophy complaints, it was reasonable to suppose that improving the circulation in the affected leg might help the ulcer to heal, and complications from a "proof" sympathectomy were unlikely. This I explained to the family, and we decided to go ahead. I next saw Hester on the operating theatre complex, and we carried out a test procedure with a local anaesthetic. Using a portable x-ray machine I inserted a long needle through Hester's back, and when I was satisfied with the position, I injected a solution of a local anaesthetic. The procedure went without problems, and afterward there were some signs of an improving circulation in the leg. The temperature went up a bit, and some colour returned. This was just sufficient to lead to the decision to carry out a definitive procedure using phenol to interrupt the sympathetic nerves permanently during a repeat admission if the first days went well. They did not. After three days the family was back in my consulting room. The pain had increased to such a level that Hester remained in bed, and hardly slept at night. Irregularities in the road surface had made the journey to the hospital unbearable.

I had (and still have) no idea what was going on here, let alone knowing what to do about it. This was neuropathic pain, and notoriously hard to treat. It was inexplicable; this does not happen after a sympathectomy, and

170

certainly not one carried out with a drug which only works for a number of hours. Here I had an 18 year old patient who was seriously incapacitated by the original trauma, and now it looked as if her life was in ruins as a result of my intervention. The only hope I could give her was that it was just a temporary exacerbation, and would settle down again. I had an awful sinking feeling in my stomach; I didn't really believe in it. Ten minutes later the father approached me alone. Until this day, I know exactly where we were standing, with him to my left side. He said, "Doctor, if it doesn't improve and Hester would rather die than go on living with this pain, will you be there for her then?" I said yes.... Under these circumstances I felt I could say nothing else, but the enormity of the possible ramifications of this left me almost in a state of shock.

Although the ulcer did eventually heal, there was no improvement in the pain, and we admitted Hester to the hospital for further evaluation with a surgical colleague. One question which continually played through my mind was: "is this pain real, or is some psychic trauma at play?"

The time came when Hester wanted euthanasia. She refused to see a psychologist; her conclusion after her sessions with the psychiatrist was that they just wouldn't take her seriously anyway. I forced her hand, saying that I was prepared to continue treating her, but only if she would submit to a psychological assessment. Euthanasia in such a situation was pretty well unthinkable, and to even countenance it without a psychological assessment would have been negligent and foolish.

In the meantime we tried to treat the pain with a series of phentolamine blocks. It involved putting a tourniquet round the upper leg, and injecting the drug into a vein with the intention of causing the contracted blood vessels to open up. It was not a very pleasant therapy to undergo when you had so much pain. Some colleagues said it was the worst thing you could do, and some believed implicitly in this treatment. But then they used to believe implicitly in blood letting with leaches; it had no beneficial effect, and nor did this.

171

The psychologist returned from his assessment with the following conclusions. Hester was quite clear in her refusal to have therapy from a psychiatrist or psychologist. He found no signs of psychopathology but concluded that she was clearly suicidal, and that it did not have the appearance of attention grabbing. She accepted that it was important to have someone to talk to, but the only person she was prepared to talk to was Dr. Jack. Oh! I felt the noose tightening round my neck.

The psychologist and I had a meeting with the psychiatrists in our hospital to decide what to do. There was not a lot of choice, and we decided that we would embark on a three-pronged plan. Although I was in no way prepared or trained, I was to talk with Hester, with the aim of helping her cope with the pain, to see whether psychic traumas were playing a role, and, basically, to keep her alive until all treatment options had been exhausted. Psychiatry was the only subject during my whole medical training that I really did well at. The psychiatrists were to be in the background to support me and help me make sense of the reports I was to write of what I was hearing. The second prong was to make sure that all reasonable treatment options had been tried and the third was to explore possibilities for euthanasia. The whole thing was so abnormal that we took the trouble to inform the inspector for mental health, and got his blessing for our plans.

In the coming months I was a frequent visitor to Hester's home. At first she lived with her parents, and after a while she moved in with a friend and her husband. A change of scenery seemed a good idea. There were always niggling doubts as to whether some traumatic event had happened in her childhood. We had many long talks, but I never found any evidence of incest or anything else significant. I can remember little of the detail of our talks. Hester obviously valued them, but I have doubts that they were useful in the long term. Hester lived in and on her bed in their living room with her guinea pig as company. She reported that she barely slept at night because of the pain, and spent much of the time listening to music. The Alan Parsons project was her favourite, and in particular "the same old sun"

Taking my life

one day at a time

Cause I can't think what else to do

Taking some time

To make up my mind

When there's no one to ask but you

The same old sun would shine in the morning

The same bright eyes would welcome me home

And the moon woud rise way over my head

And get through the night alone

Music is a powerful way to recall events and feelings, and I am playing this
CD as I write. The sadness of that time comes flooding back. Although I
never felt guilty, one thing was clear: after my intervention with the sympathectomy, her life changed from bad to intolerable. She was stuck in bed,
and I could see no sign that she would ever get out of it again. And I
wanted so much to make things better — to make amends, as it were.

During my visits we did not just talk; I tried to get her to mobilise and walk
short distances, and I got her out the house by taking her for rides in a
wheel chair. These efforts were well meant, but we were never really getting
anywhere.

It wasn't just Hester suffering; my family, friends and colleagues could see
the heavy emotional toll it was taking on me. On top of a busy full time job
with frequent on call duties I tried to be a father and husband, but there
was no day without Hester.

What was I to do? How could I extricate myself from this? Where would I
find a colleague who would want to take on such a "lost case"? And even if
I did, what then of my promise to stand by her? That felt so like betrayal,
and I knew that Hester would have been devastated. I was also preparing
documents to lay a foundation for euthanasia, which seemed ever more
likely, and terrifying from a legal point of view. And all the while Hester just

wanted to die because the pain was intolerable and she saw no future for herself.

To give her a change of scenery, she came to stay for a couple of weekends with my family; with painkillers and sedatives for the journey of about twenty minutes. I can still picture her now, thin and delicate as a bird, sitting in our living room, leg up on the sofa, playing chess with my son. These were moments when she was able to concentrate on something other than the pain, and it did so much good to see her laughing.

I looked for projects to distract Hester and give her some moments of happiness. She wanted to go to a zoo, but this seemed unattainable. One day my oldest son came home with five chicks, just hatched out at a friend's farm. I shall not forget the sight of Hester holding a little feathery bundle to her cheek.

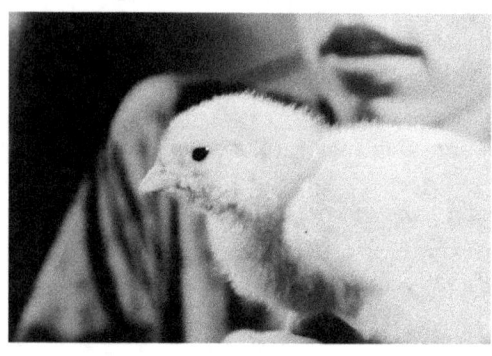

On two occasions we went to the Hoge Veluwe, a nature reserve. These were about the only times in more than a year that she came outside her own home and street and into nature. On one occasion it rained, and she sat on a rug under a plastic sheet rigged up as a shelter. Anyone else would have considered that afternoon as a dismal failure. For Hester it was perhaps one of the happiest moments of her last year. I still have a photo; a fragile Hester sitting on a blanket in the middel of a clearing in the woods enjoying a moment of relative happiness.

I felt inextricably locked into the situation.

We continued to look for treatment possibilities. We sent her to a centre where an epidural electrode was implanted into her back, next to the spinal cord. Stimulating this electrode gave some pain reduction, but after a few

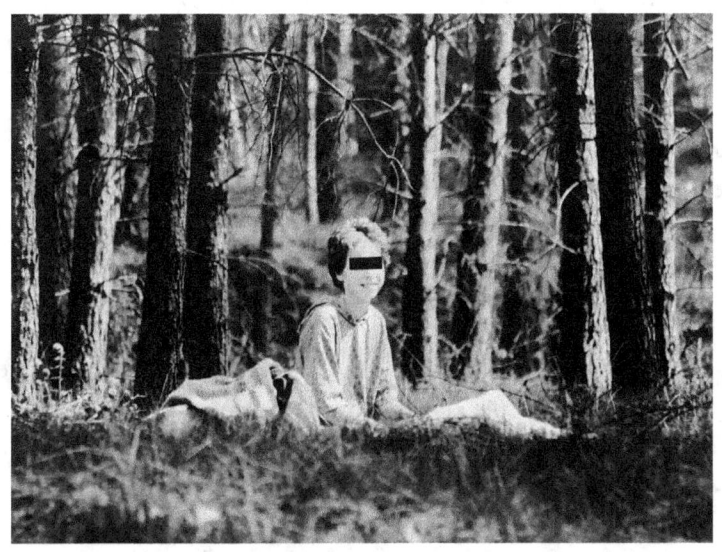

weeks it shifted its position, and had to be replaced. When it happened a second time, I realised that this would not be a long term solution for such a young woman. We then sent her to a surgeon at the university hospital in Nijmegen. This professor had a special interest in dystrophy patients, and his conclusion was that the leg should be amputated.

I knew that it was possible that in the meantime the pain sensation could be coming from a centre in the spinal cord, and that removing the leg would not only be traumatic, but might leave the pain unchanged. At this time Hester was lying in our intensive care department with continuous infusions of powerful painkillers and sedatives. I decided to carry out nerve blocks of the sciatic and femoral nerves. If the pain remained unaltered after these blocks, then it was certain that amputating the leg would offer no solution to her problems. So we carried out the blocks, and Hester reported that the leg was now numb, but that the pain was as bad as ever.

By then, most of my colleagues and the nursing staff were convinced that Hester was not suffering from real pain, but from "conversion," something we used to call hysteria. Although I was never able to fully exclude this from my thoughts, I still had a gut feeling that the pain was real, and now

175

the only explanation left over was that a centre had evolved in the spinal cord which was maintaining and amplifying the pain. I was aware of this possibility, but had never been confronted with it. To test it, I sedated Hester in the operating theatre, placed a catheter in the spinal fluid, and injected a small amount of local anaesthetic. We took her back to the intensive care department, and when she woke, she reported that she could not feel the lower half of her body, and that the pain was unchanged. I realised that this confirmed the diagnosis of conversion, in line with the opinion of colleagues and nursing staff and I felt thoroughly disillusioned.

I spent some time deep in thought, and then another possibility came to mind. What if there was a spinal pain generating centre, and it was at a higher level than the catheter tip I had placed? I found myself unable to give up on this, and we went back to the operating theatre. We put Hester into a light sleep, placed the catheter tip a few centimeters higher, and injected a small dose of local anaesthetic. Hester collapsed suddenly and dramatically: her breathing stopped, and the blood pressure dropped steeply. I really thought that we were going to lose her.

(Side note: Hester wanted to die, and there I was, terribly close to granting her wish. And yet as a doctor it was unthinkable that I could let her go as a complication of a treatment. The doctor's ego saves a life against the wishes of the patient! What should I think of this?)

I could only think of one possible cause of the collapse. Hester was on high doses of opiate painkillers. In these doses they would normally cause serious depression of the central nervous system. In someone with severe pain, the depression is countered by the stimulation caused by the pain. If you suddenly removed the pain the opiates would have a "free hand" and the patient could collapse! I became excited; if this were to be the case, then we had proved that the pain was genuine. There was one conclusive way to demonstrate this further and that was to administer a drug that would (partially) reverse the effects of the opiates, and see what happened. So we gave a dose of Naloxone, an opiate antagonist. The effect was miraculous; within two minutes, Hester woke up, and with a broad smile said that the pain was gone.

176

This was a watershed moment in my thinking. The process had taken place while Hester was asleep, and there was no way I could explain this through conversion: from then on I was convinced that I was dealing with a rare and exceptionally severe chronic pain syndrome.

The joy was short-lived. We infused a local anaesthetic with a pump into the spinal catheter; at first it worked, but then tachyphylaxis set in. This is common with local anaesthetic drugs; they become less effective with continuous use. Apart from that, I realised that it was unrealistic to think that we could keep a catheter in her spinal space for the rest of her life; at some point infection would set in.

We were running out of treatment options quickly, and euthanasia seemed the only way forward. (Forward???)

At that time in the Netherlands, euthanasia had just become legally possible for terminally ill patients, as long as certain criteria had been satisfied. An 18 year old girl with chronic pain was an entirely different category, and there was no precedent for this. In Rotterdam there was a well known professor of psychology, who had done a great deal for the development of lawmaking around euthanasia, and he had set up a group with an ethicist and a GP to assist in difficult cases. (This man has done many good things, and helped me at a very difficult time; I was very saddened to learn that he had to give up his post after a plagiarism case. Does this have anything to do with the chapter on ambition?)

I approached him, and he was sympathetic; he asked me to send him all the details I had, and then invited me to Rotterdam for a meeting of his euthanasia team. After we had gone through all the information, the conclusion was that I should help Hester by carrying of euthanasia if no solution to her pain could be found. I was advised to take the first step of approaching a psychiatrist in Nijmegen who was sympathetic to euthanasia, and could be asked to examine Hester to confirm that there was no psychopathology which might complicate the situation further. I phoned the psychiatrist, who reacted as if he had been stung by a bee. "No thank you very much, I am already being investigated by the ministry of justice for a similar case". These were early days for euthanasia, even in the Nether-lands, and the legal ramifications were not yet clarified. Eventually I man-aged to make an appointment with another psychiatrist, and after a mighty struggle persuaded Hester to make the trip to Nijmegen. I was later dis-gusted to find that the psychiatrist had left the assessment to a doctor in training. However, the conclusion was that there was no evident psy-chopathology. That was one hurdle taken. At the same time I approached a lawyer who was at the forefront of euthanasia jurisprudence. Having stud-ied the whole case he thought that I might "get away with it," but that it would be a close call. Not very encouraging!

The next step was to look for somebody of high status who could confirm that all reasonable treatment options had been tried. I wrote to Dr S, one of the most respected pain specialists in the Netherlands, explaining all we had done, and the euthanasia request. I received a letter back in which he confirmed that there were no other treatment options, and added as an af-terthought, "But this may never be a reason to carry out euthanasia" that last phrase angers me to this day. One thing I did not need in this precari-ous situation was to have to face a judge with this letter in his hands! Hes-ter's GP was of no support at any time. It was he who had missed the diag-nosis and sent Hester to the psychiatrist, and after that he distanced himself from the case.

My direct colleagues and my hospital psychiatrists were supportive and kind, and yet in general I felt very alone in this period. I knew what I had to do, and I was scared; not of the act of euthanasia itself, but for myself and all the consequences that may follow. I had a good career, and a family to support. What if I was struck off the Medical register? Looking back I feel shame; shame that I did not have the guts to do what I believed was right and face the consequences.

Hester became more impatient, and I kept on trying to find support. I had the explicit support of the psychologist's committee, but Hester's GP didn't want to know anything about it, and no one else was prepared to stick their neck out (this was understandable — even these days when euthanasia is an accepted practice in the Netherlands this would be a difficult case; back then it was more or less unthinkable). While all this was going on, we implanted a port under the skin in her chest, to which we connected a pump with morphine.

One step I had taken was for Hester to sign a living testament in which she declared that she refused all therapy except for symptomatic measures, and eventually this proved to be the key to a solution. It meant that we were prohibited from giving any treatment not directed at her pain symptoms.

When it became clear that there was no other way out, I contacted the inspector of health by phone, and explained the situation. Having heard it all, he said, "It looks as if you have no choice here, so go ahead". Relief! But short-lived: within an hour he rang me back, and said that he had discussed it with the public prosecutor, and that I should certainly be prosecuted. He then asked me (and his words are burned forever in my mind, "Can she not do it herself? By stopping eating, or jumping off a building?" I was furious, and said, "Is that your idea of being a doctor?" The precariously balanced foundation of support was crumbling. My heart sank; what now?

One night, at about three a.m. the phone rang. It was Hester's friend, ringing to tell me that Hester had just injected 300 mg of morphine directly into the port, and thus straight into the bloodstream. A normal dose of this painkiller after an operation would be ten milligrams, so this was a massive overdose. It would have killed anyone not habituated to the drug. Admitting Hester to the hospital as an emergency would have been in contravention to her living testament, and as such illegal, so I went straight to her home, and found her sitting in bed, clear as a bell, and complaining that the pain was worse than ever. I rang the GP to ask if he would back me up if I injected more, and it proved lethal. He wanted nothing to do with it. I did not do it, which I think in retrospect was cowardly. It would certainly have hit the national headlines: "doctor injects twenty year old with lethal dose of morphine; arrested by police".

The next day Hester started to run a high temperature, and I was sure that she had introduced bacteria into her bloodstream. I admitted her to the hospital, with the promise that I would abide by her testament, and just give

179

her symptomatic treatment, but no antibiotics. My anaesthesia colleagues were marvellous, and took the last steps out of my hands. We gave no treatment for the septicaemia (infection of the bloodstream), and just ran infusions of painkillers and sedatives. Hester's family knew what was happening, and were with her to the end. She died after a few seemingly interminable days.

At that time people who had died were usually kept at a funeral parlour until the funeral took place. However I knew that some were taken home so that the family could be at their side whenever they wished. When I suggested this, her family was open to the idea, and Hester spent the days before the funeral in a chilled and open coffin in their home. This was good, and allowed her parents and sisters to say good bye in their own way; I remember pictures of butterflies in the coffin.

I attended the funeral, and gave my last respects for Hester in a speech during the service.

I now look back over more than thirty years, and still don't know what to make of it all. Important questions remain, and for some I have tentative answers. Was my behaviour unprofessional? Yes, it certainly was. I came to care deeply for this girl. Should I feel badly about this? Did I harm her in any way? No, I don't think so; I gave her what I could, I brought a little sunshine into her dark life, and did everything within my power to treat her. Is it possible that I came to mean so much to her that getting better was no option because then she would lose me? It niggles at the back of my mind sometimes, but knowing that I had taken all possible steps in her diagnosis and treatment, softens this concern somewhat.

I often think how I could have done things differently, and what I would advise another colleague to do in the same situation. Probably the most controversial step was in becoming her "therapist" with no formal training. But even here, this step was only taken after consulting with psychologist, psychiatrist and inspector while the alternative was to let her put an end to her own life in her own way. Bitter enough for me is have to admit that in the end that's just what she did. That still makes me feel ashamed - I left

180

her to sort it out herself because I was afraid for my own skin. Looking back now I just don't know what I should have done otherwise, and really wouldn't know how to advise another in a similar situation. R.I.P. Hester.

Take home message

God only knows!

I can calculate the motion of heavenly bodies, but not the madness of people.

Sir Isaac Newton

Will you help me die?

Euthanasia is a subject that many doctors will be confronted with during their career, and many of them will find it very hard to cope with. It is emotionally charged, and has complicated moral and ethical considerations. Writing this chapter was the greatest challenge of this book, but it is important that every doctor is able to form an opinion, and decide whether they can or cannot support euthanasia. The aim of this chapter is to help the reader get a clearer idea of the issues, and to be able to make an informed choice if and when confronted with such situations. The next chapter presents a bitter-sweet account of euthanasia for a young woman with cancer.

One factor that makes euthanasia such a difficult subject is that religious beliefs colour the perspective and influence decisions. That may at first seem fine to believers, but there is one great problem. The foundations on which religious beliefs are built are often vague and it is then not surprising that the beliefs themselves are often a matter of interpretation. Interpretations vary enormously in time and between religions: is circumcision necessary? Does a blood transfusion block the path to heaven or not? Is anticonception forbidden or acceptable in the eyes of God? Is female genital mutilation a necessary act or a crime? May meat only be eaten if the beast is slaughtered in the appropriate way, or does that not matter? Is riding your bicycle on a Sunday a sin? Is euthanasia acceptable under certain circumstances, or never? A follower of one religious denomination will believe quite different things to someone from another.

It is not my intention to make the reader uncomfortable, but to demonstrate the complexity of this matter. A doctor working in a society in which everyone has the same convictions will not have a problem, but more and more we live in a multicultural setting. Basing one's medical practice on the beliefs of one particular religion is in effect disrespecting the beliefs of all the other religions and the beliefs of atheists. In an ideal situation, we doctors would use more objective criteria and arguments when deciding matters like euthanasia. This remains a utopia because doctors also have their own religious convictions, which need to be respected just as much as those of the patients.

"Objective criteria" makes it sound simple, and sometimes it is. If you vaccinate a sufficient portion of the population, then some devastating diseases can be eradicated. Smallpox is a perfect example. It now only survives in a very secure laboratory setting. Allowing religious beliefs to influence medical decisions is the reason that polio still exists and causes serious illness outside the laboratory. If you think that that is a clear-cut reason to vaccinate everyone, some religious people would disagree — to them, if you get polio, that is the will of God.

Here is another example, which seems at first sight simpler, and may look like a digression. Last week I worked with a plastic surgeon. One of his cases was a young woman for a breast enlargement operation. When she was under the anaesthetic, and the sheets were removed, we were looking at a beautifully proportioned body. I asked the surgeon whether he thought putting in two 500 mL prosthetics would be an improvement. "It's going to be ugly," he replied. "Then why are you doing it?" "Because she thinks that it is going to be beautiful, and I have to follow her judgement, not mine." "So what would you do if she asked you to place 600 mL prosthetics?" "Oh, I wouldn't do that." Think about that for a moment. What he was saying, in effect, is that it was the patient's judgement until he felt so uncomfortable with it that he could no longer put his own belief aside. Then he switches to his own judgement. Some of his colleagues would have switched directly, refusing to carry out the operation at all, and some would happily place the 600 mL protheses. Who is right and who is wrong here? I felt that I was complicit in deforming a human body, but of course that is my judgement; is it more valid than that of the patient? The point I want to make is that even when medical decisions seem simple, they are often not.

184

The situation with euthanasia is in a way similar. Some colleagues would refuse such a request outright, some would agree to a form of terminal sedation, and some would be prepared to honour the request fully. Again, there is no right or wrong, just as there is no right or wrong in the request itself, outside the religious context.

The international declaration of human rights gives us the right to self-determination. This implies that I have the right to put an end to my life when I no longer see a reason to live, or when the quality of my life has been brought down by illness to a level that I judge that being alive is no longer worth the price I have to pay for it — be it mental or physical suffering. Note that I write, I judge, and no one else.

However, in the UK, and many other countries, if a patient reaches that point, and the doctor helps them terminate their suffering, no matter how well motivated or understandable, then the doctor will be criminally liable. Despite euthanasia being illegal, it does happen, even in those countries where it is forbidden by law; however not having a legal framework has very serious negative consequences.

1. Because it is done secretly, there is no check on how often it is happening.

2. There are no guidelines for doctors as to how the situation should be approached.

3. It has to be done in the dark, excluding colleagues from supervising and helping evaluate the psychological situation of the patient, the indications and other possible treatment options.

4. There is no way of knowing whether the most effective drugs are being used.

5. There is no national registration of euthanasia.

6. Euthanasia is not reported to the authorities: so there are no checks and balances possible.

Compare this to the Dutch system, where each case has to reported and evaluated. A second doctor has to be consulted, and there are many other guidelines to ensure that the procedure was justified and carried out in accordance with the regulations. Cases in which the doctor has not followed guidelines are investigated and where necessary prosecuted. There is no carte blanche in the Netherlands. Doctors no longer have to carry the procedure out as a crime that has to be hidden, but can do it openly, in the presence of the family. Society is looking over their shoulders, and there is transparency about numbers and indications. Fears about the slippery slope and the society becoming less caring are simply not born out by the facts. The Dutch situation is used by many in the UK to demonstrate for and against euthanasia. I am convinced that looking objectively at the facts instead of fear-mongering shows that it is a system which, although not perfect, is far and away more honest and effective than what is happening in most countries of the world.

If people choose to believe, for whatever reason, that euthanasia is wrong, and they want nothing to do with it, then that is their good right; they will neither ask for it, nor carry it out. The UK is a democracy, a secular state and a country in which the majority support euthanasia. Yet the opponents, although in the minority, have sufficient power to impose their beliefs on the majority, believers and non-believers alike. This is not democracy. The situation in the UK is not unique.

I do not wish to get into all the arguments for and against euthanasia, but the two religious objections most heard are: life is a gift from God, and suffering brings you closer to God. Because life is a gift from God, then only God can take it away. It is not immediately obvious to me why the first and second part of this argument are automatically coupled, but that is the argument.

The idea that suffering is good for our spiritual growth, and must not be curtailed is rather vague. For instance, is all suffering valuable? If so, the

186

whole medical profession could be done away with, as preventing suffering is their main reason for existing. Is a hip replacement done to relieve painful arthritis acceptable? Or will that stunt our spiritual growth? Is reducing terminal suffering by giving ample doses of painkillers also wrong? As with so many of these arguments, their believability rests on their vagueness. Drill down too deep, and they fall apart.

The catholic church claims that people who ask for euthanasia are not really asking for it — they are asking for attention, love and care. This is possibly true in some cases, and certainly untrue in others. Some people have reached a stage where they just want to die. The church also says that doctors granting such patients their wish is not compatible with good patient care. To my mind, for patients in such a situation it is the last bit of really good care a doctor can give.

It is clearly a good thing for society to take measures to prevent people killing others, and yet society is quite capable of generating laws to create exceptions which allow adequate protection of life without prohibiting someone from asking a doctor to help them exercise their right to self-determination. The Netherlands has demonstrated this.

In my practice I have been confronted with Jehovah's witnesses who were prepared to let their children die rather than allowing a life-saving blood transfusion. I invited them into my home in order to try to understand the basis for a belief so strong that they were prepared to die for it, and to let their children die. What it really boiled down to, was the bible stating, "Thou shalt not partake of blood". As an anaesthetist, I found these arguments unconvincing. However, if an adult refused a blood transfusion, I felt that that was within their right to self-determination, even if their arguments made no sense to me. I had one patient on the recovery ward who had lost so much blood that she probably would not survive. I left the choice to her, and she decided to have the blood transfusion as long as it was given on the theatre complex. She also desired a new, clean infusion system before returning to the ward so that visitors would not see what had happened. What I was not prepared to do was to let a child die for the

187

same reasons, and in such cases we had to obtain a temporary injunction from a judge in order to give a transfusion.

The strange thing in countries prohibiting euthanasia is that it seems to be acceptable for religion to cause death: if you refuse to vaccinate your child and he dies of measles, there will be no legal consequences. If you, as a doctor, respect the wish of a terminal patient to die, then you are a criminal. Many will say, "That's quite different". They will be right: the child did not ask to die, the terminal patient did.

In fairness it must be said that religious objections are not the only arguments against euthanasia, but I am certain that if it were not for the church, common sense would have prevailed long ago.

Well, the arguments go on and on, and I am glad to be working in the Netherlands, where the will of the great majority has been respected by medical authorities, politicians and the mainline churches. The Netherlands has had the courage to accept and admit that euthanasia actually happens, has always happened, and needs regulating to ensure that it is carried out at the right time by the right people for the right reasons and in the right way.

To put it rather crudely, the UK settles for exporting this difficult problem to Switzerland, rather like Ireland exported abortion to the UK, until eventually the law was changed. I presume that this will someday happen with euthanasia, but it seems far away at present.

In 1995 I read that a film about euthanasia in the Netherlands was to be shown on the BBC. It followed a Dutch GP and a patient with terminal ALS who had requested euthanasia. When I heard that the BBC was to be broadcasting it, I realised the commotion it would cause in the UK and that opponents of euthanasia would use the documentary to make the Dutch system look bad. So I phoned the BBC, and said, "I am sure that there will be discussion programmes after this broadcast, and what you need is a British doctor who works in the Netherlands, has carried out euthanasia under the Dutch system, and actually knows what he is talking about". They were apologetic, but the discussion programmes were already filled. About

188

an hour later the phone went, and it was the BBC; would I be prepared to fly over to London at short notice to take part in a panel discussion? You bet I would!

This was incidentally the one and only occasion in my life when I felt like a VIP. I was flown to London, and waiting for me was a chauffeur with a board on a stick, "Dr. Jack BBC," and a large Mercedes that brought me to broadcasting house. There I was rushed through the makeup department to cover the worse blemishes, and into the TV studio.

The discussion was led by the well known journalist, Michael Ignatius, and arguing against euthanasia were Dame Cicely Courtney, who was a delightful lady, and one of those responsible for setting up hospices in the UK, a hospice doctor and a journalist. Arguing the case for euthanasia were sir Ludovic Kennedy, at that time vice-president of the voluntary euthanasia society, the Dutch doctor Van Ooijen who had carried out the euthanasia, and myself.

I am sure Cicely Courtney genuinely cared for her patients. I think that she really believed that once a patient discovered what a hospice had to offer, they would no longer want euthanasia. And there is some truth to this; I am sure that many patients are frightened to die, or just not ready, and that optimal end of life care will be of enormous value to them. She and Kennedy commanded respect. One statement from Kennedy which has remained with me was, "My mother wanted to die: she was not interested in hospice care — she just wanted to die".

The main argument from those opposed to euthanasia is that it is never necessary if optimal terminal care is offered. What this comes down to, is that at the moment that I would give euthanasia, they will sedate the patient to the point that they no longer suffer until they die.

So this gives rise to the question "what is euthanasia?" If I give a patient an intravenous infusion of normal saline, and add some morphine so that the patient is sedated, and gradually increase the dose, so that the patient dies after three days, that is "terminal sedation". It is legal in the UK, and the doctor can go home to a well earned dinner. If he gives the same infusion, and injects a drug so that the patient dies ten minutes later, that is euthanasia, and the doctor goes to a well earned jail sentence. So what if the patient dies after 24 hours of this infusion, or 36 hours, or 12 hours? Is that terminal sedation or euthanasia? The intention is the same; the end result is the same, the only difference is in time. Is that a reason to allow the one, and forbid the other? I don't think so. We need more nuanced thinking than that.

If you believe that the suffering is necessary, as some in the church do, then "terminal sedation" as it is called is surely just as "wrong". The hypocritical thing is that although in both situations doctors know that the end is nigh, and want to alleviate suffering, the one pretends that sedating the patient with morphine is not hastening their death, when in fact it is just watered down euthanasia.

I do not want to sound too critical of British doctors here; they have to do the best they can for their patients within the constraints allowed by law. And many of them will be as frustrated with this law as I am. I have been in this same situation before legislation in the Netherlands was changed and I too carried out euthanasia under another name.

I am also not saying that there is no place for what is often called "terminal sedation". If a patient wants it that way, for religious or other reasons, then I have no objection.

In my view a doctor, and preferably the patient's own doctor, should carry out the euthanasia. Some consider this to be in contravention to the first line of the Hippocratic oath taken by all doctors, "primum non nocere " (in the first place, do no harm). As I see it, we are doing harm to a patient who is suffering and wants to die when we *refuse* the request.

My contribution to the television debate was to demonstrate the hypocrisy of the UK position, and to defend the Dutch system. Ignatius picked up on this, and tried to press the opponents of euthanasia on the matter, without success. They were evasive about it and on the question of whether there

190

could ever be justification for euthanasia. Philips was so concerned about the effects of legalisation undermining society, that she felt that the individual's interests had to be subservient to that. In the twenty years that followed this discussion, there is no evidence to think that Dutch society has become less caring, nor that misuse of euthanasia has become a problem.

If I compare the Dutch and UK systems, there are differences which make it clear to me that someday the UK will be obliged to change the law. They have been talking about it for more than twenty years, and are essentially no further.

First of all, is euthanasia being carried out in the UK? If so, how often, how well performed, how well motivated and documented? For the first question, the answer is clearly yes. Caring doctors will alleviate patient's suffering as well as they can, and that sometimes means shortening life. For the other questions, in the UK we have no idea; doctors are not silly enough to admit to breaking the law, so euthanasia is not carried out, and not documented. There is thus no way of knowing how well motivated it is, nor how well it is carried out.

I shall never forget the first time I performed euthanasia in the Netherlands, before it was legalised. An elderly lady had requested it, and I was asked by the physician if I would consider carrying it out. It was a clear-cut case of a terminal illness in a patient who had just had enough. I carried out her wishes in secret, injecting a lethal combination of drugs that would enable her to sleep, and then stop breathing. I made no record of what I had done, and was terrified that I would be found out and punished.

Three years later I was approached by a nurse, who told me that she had cared for that woman for months, and was so hurt that she was excluded from the last act. I explained why, and she understood, but of course it was a completely unsatisfactory situation, and I felt bad, despite standing by my decision to help the patient. The family knew and respected her wishes, according to the patient, but I never spoke to them, and they would have to take this secret with them to their own graves to avoid getting me into

191

trouble. Just imagine it, your loved one has undergone euthanasia, and this emotional event may not be spoken of. That is how it is in the UK today.

Compare that with how things went after the law was changed. Then I could discuss it openly with family and medical and nursing staff. I could get a second physician, preferably a psychiatrist, to see that the patient was of sound mind; I could make an appointment so that family could be there with the patient until the end. The family are now free to talk about it if they wish, and I can, and must, keep an accurate record of why and how the euthanasia was carried out. After the death of the patient I report the euthanasia to the coroner, and the case is judged by a regional committee. Six weeks after my first euthanasia under the new law I found a letter on my desk, which I nervously opened, to learn that I would not be prosecuted. If this death had been in the grey area, such as a malformed baby, or a psychiatric case, then it could be that a test case would be held. But even then, if my motivation was clear and the procedure correct, I should have nothing to fear. This is how jurisprudence is built up, and euthanasia given its rightful place in society.

The UK chooses to keep it illegal, so that although we know that it's done, that is all we know.

Some are afraid of the "slippery slope" argument: that once you legalise it, it will get out of hand. As proof, these people show how in the Netherlands the number of euthanasia cases has risen drastically since it was legalised. Well, of course it has! Doctors now report what they previously kept hidden. But I am convinced that the vast majority of these reported cases are legitimate, otherwise they would simply not get reported. In the beginning of this new phase many doctors were frightened to report euthanasia until they saw that it was safe to do so, and even today some are still wary, and prefer the old way of doing things, which I think a great pity. The braver ones went first.

Is there malpractice in euthanasia in the Netherlands? Maybe, but that has nothing to do with legalisation, because malpractice will not be reported.

And in the UK? It's just as likely or unlikely. These malpractice cases have nothing to do with the legalisation issue.

Apart from these arguments, there is the matter of how the euthanasia is carried out. For this reason as well, patients in the Netherlands are far better off than in the UK. Where euthanasia has to be carried out in secret, it is very often done with an overdose of morphine.

I remember well one old man who had been on an infusion of morphine for a week or so; he was terminal, and ready to die. It was in the time that euthanasia would have been legally possible, but the physician was wary of doing this, and thus just kept raising the morphine dose. However, when someone has had morphine for some time, they become very resistant to its effects (as was the case with Hester, who's story is presented in another chapter). The old man's wife wanted to be with him at the end, so she sat next to him, and only left his side when she was exhausted and just had to sleep. You guessed it — she had hardly left the room, when he died alone. I found that such a shame for her, and it was not necessary. In the UK that will be the most used method, and it is eventually successful but unpredictable. The alternative in the UK would be that a fast working drug is administered whilst nervously looking round in case you are caught out.

There is a much more elegant alternative which I used once euthanasia was legalised. To start with, it means making an appointment with the patient, which is a bit surreal the first time. "When do you want to die?" Usually the answer is as soon as possible, once the necessary procedures have been completed, and the family are available. I used two infusion pumps, the first with a hypnotic drug, which we use when we give a general anaesthetic. I set this pump running so that the patient gradually falls asleep over a period of about five minutes. When they sleep, the second pump is started with a mixture of a muscle relaxant and a very powerful synthetic form of morphine. The effect of these two drugs is that the patient's breathing becomes gradually slower and more superficial until it stops. This gives what looks to the family like a completely natural and peaceful death. It can also be timed so that it lasts for whatever period seems best. Time for the family to see a 'natural' death, but not endless. It requires courage to do it openly, but my

193

standpoint is clear: if the patient and the doctor have both decided that euthanasia is indicated and wished for, just do it, in the most elegant way possible.

Euthanasia for psychiatric patients and dementia

These are two groups of patients that I find particularly difficult, and for two different reasons.

There can be no doubt that a psychiatric patient's suffering can be just as severe as that of a cancer patient. There is one major difference: the cancer patient's suffering is limited in time, whereas that of the psychiatric patient's pain can go on for a lifetime. There is no doubt in my mind that for some of these patients, life is a living hell, and euthanasia could be just as justified as in a cancer patient. The difficulty is in finding objective proof that the situation will not improve. Euthanasia is occasionally carried out for psychiatric patients in the Netherlands. The situation then is usually a patient who has been asking to be allowed to die for years, and for whom no therapy has worked. I am just glad that I have never been confronted with it.

Dementia is also a very difficult issue. There are many people, including myself, who state unequivocally that if they are no longer able te make their own decisions through cognitive decline, then they want euthanasia. The problem is that once they have arrived at that point they are often no longer able to clearly state their wishes. It makes some difference if there is a previously written living will, but even then the question arises as to whether the person has changed their mind in the light of their changed circumstances. At the time of writing a doctor is being prosecuted in the Netherlands for carrying out euthanasia on a patient who had always been clear and consistent in her wish no longer to live if she became dement. When it came to the last period of her life, in which dementia was playing an increasing role, she sometimes did, and sometimes did not want euthanasia. When the doctor came to carry it out, with the family present, they first had to sedate the patient, and then hold her down while the euthanasia was performed. This is obviously a highly contentious situation, even though the intention was obviously sincere. These are the borderline cases and the

194

Dutch justice system then steps in to try to define the acceptable limits. However, it is no simple situation, and it is a fact that dementia is one of the main reasons for requesting euthanasia, and at the same the situation in which doctors very often feel unable to carry out the previously so clearly stipulated request. What it boils down to, is that you are either not dement enough, or too dement for euthanasia to be straightforward. There is a trend developing in the Netherlands to make short video clips of patients with early dementia. They often have lucid moments, and these can be captured, and presented to the doctor to make clear that it is still the clear unequivocal wish of the person. I know of no other good answer to this, and I just hope that I, and my family and doctors may be spared ever being confronted with it.

Take home message

A doctor is often confronted with moral and ethical decisions. Realising how complicated these can be will help you to be more understanding of others — patients and colleagues — and help inform your decisions when confronted with such a request.

From euthanasia to pancakes

This last chapter is an example of how tragedy and beauty can go hand in hand with euthanasia.

Jolanda was twenty-two years old when she got married. I have seen photographs of her on her wedding day; radiant with a luxuriant mass of long dark brown hair and a red dress. This dress, however, had to be let out at the seams at the last minute because it didn't fit round the waist any more. Her abdomen felt a little blown up, and she went to the GP who diagnosed irritable bowels, and gave her a laxative.

I met Jolanda two years later. Gone, the lovely hair and the full healthy face. The body wasted. By the time her GP had sent her to a specialist, she was found to have ovarian cancer. A laparotomy was performed, and the tumour was seen to be disseminated, and inoperable. Chemotherapy had done its work on her hair, but little to cure her. Inside that sick body was a women full of life and energy who just wanted to live, and knew she had to die.

I arrived at the flat she shared with her husband, asked by her oncologist to see if I could do anything to help relieve her pain. This was just a few years after my traumatic experience with Hester, and I had pledged myself not to get so involved with patients again. There was one crucial difference which made it possible for me say yes to the oncologist; it was clear that this was going to be a short-lived contact, literally.

196

Jolanda lay on a bed in their small flat, opposite a window looking out onto a balcony. From the bed she had no view. She was in a lot of pain, and had side effects from the drugs. I suggested that we could place a spinal catheter and a morphine pump, which would deliver morphine directly to the spinal cord, and probably control her pain to some extent. I said that we should need to admit her to the hospital to do this, but she would refused outright. She'd had enough of hospitals, and bad doctors, and bad treatments.

At that moment I could have dropped the case, but I didn't. I pointed out the risks of infection if I were to place the catheter at home (probably incorrectly — if the procedure is carried out with sterile precautions, then the home environment is probably safer than a hospital with all its resistant bacteria). I left it with her and her husband to think about, and at the next visit they asked me to carry out the procedure at home. It was simple enough and I did it with an assistant who was prepared to join me in this unusual project.

The result was good: improved pain control with fewer side effects. During one of my visits to check on the spinal catheter, Jolanda asked me if I would be prepared to carry out euthanasia if she wanted it in the future. I had no problem saying yes to this — she had a terminal illness, and I felt that she had the right to decide when she had had enough. Her major worry was that she had been warned that a fistula could develop between the stomach and the lower gut, causing her to vomit faeces. She saw no reason to prolong life further if that were to occur.

Jolanda was at that time certainly not ready to die. A month before I met her, she had realised an ambition. She was the vocalist in a pop band until she became ill, and had always wanted to make a recording. This she did a few months before she died. I have a video of the making of the recordings, together with her two sisters and the backing group. It is unbelievable how much power and energy came through that emaciated body! Her face was thin, and her head bald, but the energy radiating from her eyes and voice made me shiver.

During my visits, she and her husband would talk about the end; I remember them agonising about the funeral. They were non-believers, but wanted a funeral of sorts. "Why don't you arrange it yourselves," I suggested, and they took this up with enthusiasm, and organised the whole thing together. Jolanda was wonderfully brave, and full of humour, and we laughed a lot together discussing the funeral arrangements. That sounds perhaps unbelievable, but humour makes the unmentionable yet accessible.

In that period, I gave lessons on the subject of euthanasia at a regional school of nursing. I asked Jolanda whether she would be prepared to come with me, and tell the nurses herself how it is to be preparing yourself to undergo euthanasia. She was immediately willing to do so. However, in the last months of her life she became weaker, and was bed-ridden, and it was no longer possible for her to come to the next lesson. As second best we made a video. Her husband operated the camera, and I interviewed Jolanda. At the end of the interview with her, we recorded briefly how it felt for her husband. He thought then that it would give no emotional problems for him; he didn't want to lose her, but realised that he was going to, and did not want her to suffer more than necessary.

I used this video for the coming years in my lessons to the nurses, and it always made a deep impression. At the end of the film you could hear a pin drop in the lecture room.

By this time Jolanda had lived in bed in that small, rather dark living room without any real view for months. I suggested that it would be good for her to get out for a change of scenery. It was winter, cold and early dark. Her husband and I managed to get her along the balcony and down the stairs in a wheel chair, and into my car. We drove to a local lake, and installed Jolanda in a beach chair with a thick blanket around her. There she sat for an hour as the sun went down, and was so happy to be able to see a sunset for perhaps the last time. We then went on to my house, where I cooked pancakes for us all, and afterward took them home again.

A little while after this Jolanda moved to her sister's house for the last part of her life. There she had more space, and light, and could be cared for

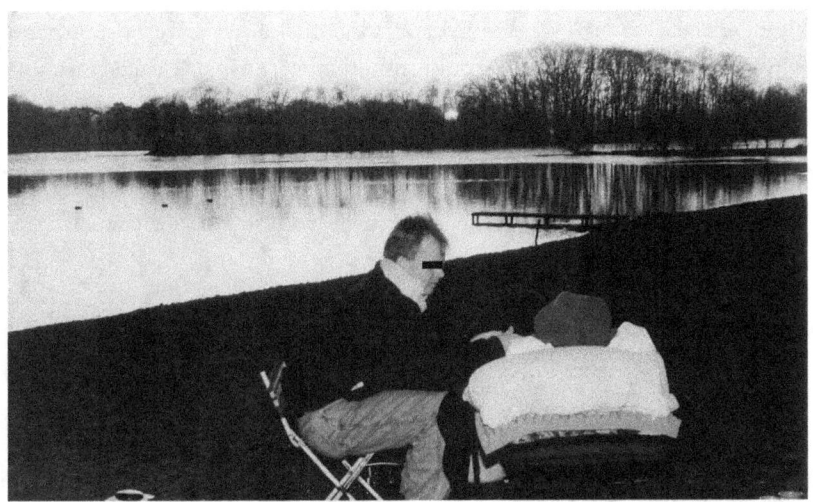

better.

Around the Christmas period of that year, Jolanda called me to say that she had vomited faeces, and was ready for euthanasia. We agreed on a date, and I remember Jolanda asking me, "What if I want to cancel it at the last minute — will that be all right?" "You have made an agreement, and you'll have to stick to it," I replied. She knew me well enough, and laughed. A day before the appointment Jolanda rang to say that she was not ready. I think that she was afraid; it was suddenly very real and final and it took another two weeks before she rang again to say that she was now fully prepared.

By this time, we had discussed the matter with the GP, who was very supportive, and a psychiatrist had assessed her as one of the obligatory formalities in the procedure. Jolanda was no ordinary patient; she had clear ideas about what she wanted; she wanted to die at home, and she wanted to die in the arms of her husband, and she didn't want to die too quickly. I can imagine that many of my colleagues would have balked at this, but I found her reasons compelling, and wanted to fulfil her last wishes to the best of my ability.

When the day came, we installed Jolanda and her husband upstairs in her sister's bed. I set up a drip, and attached two pumps which I had borrowed (without permission) from the hospital, and started the first at a slow rate. I asked her husband to give a call downstairs when she fell asleep, and joined the waiting family. After about twenty minutes her husband called me upstairs. I went into the room, and there was Jolanda sitting up in bed! "Nigel," she said, "I'm hungry! I can't go to heaven if I'm hungry, can I?" "No," I replied, "you have no idea of the opening times up there". "You once made a pancake for me" she went on, "will you make one for me now?" This euthanasia was getting like Alice in wonderland.

I went to the kitchen, and together with her sister made a pancake. Jolanda, who had barely eaten anything in the past weeks, ate it up with relish.

"Are you ready now?" She was ready. "I'm going to set the pump a bit faster now, because before you know it, you'll be ordering a five course meal!" With a smile, Jolanda fell asleep, and was dead twenty minutes later.

At her funeral, her band played for her, and I played the piano and made a short speech.

Jolanda's husband met one of my sons on the train about a year later, and said that he felt guilty at having assisted in the death of his wife. I invited him round to my house, and really only a short talk was necessary. I asked him if Jolanda would have died soon anyway, which was an obvious yes, and what her wishes were. "To die in my arms" "And you gave her that? Could you possibly have done anything else?" I think this made it easier for him. Years later he told me he was well and re-married.

This may sound strange to many, but as I look back over the years, this remains an experience I treasure. A lovely person died, and that was tragic, but I was privileged to know her, and able to give her the best possible end to her life. More than that was not mine to give.

The great French marshall Lyautey once asked his gardener to plant a tree. The gardener objected that the tree was slow growing and would not reach maturity for 100 years. The marshall replied, "In that case there is no time to lose; plant it this afternoon!"

John F. Kennedy

Author information

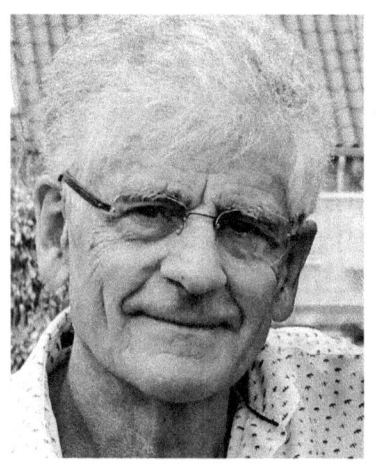

Nigel Jack was born in England in 1947. He studied medicine at the University of St Andrews in Scotland, qualifying in 1972 and worked for two years in Perth Royal Infirmary. He then travelled with his wife and 2 young children to Chingola, Zambia where he was medical officer for one of the copper mine corporations. There he was gynaecologist, anaesthetist, physician, paediatrician etc. rotating from one function to the next, and he pitied his patients for having no one more experienced. He returned to Canterbury, England in 1974 and trained as anaesthetist and became a fellow of the faculty of anaesthetists of the Royal College of Surgeons in 1977. In that year he moved with his Dutch wife and two boys to the Netherlands, where he worked for more than 40 years before retiring in 2019. He has always had a passionate interest in psychology and communication, and completed courses in NLP and mediation, both of which he considers formative and of great personal value.